JUDGES' CITATION

Grace Talusan has written a remarkable memoir in *The Body Papers*, training an unflinching eye on the most delicate and fraught contours of her own life as an immigrant and survivor of trauma and illness. She tackles with literary subtlety and a deep reservoir of compassion the paradoxes imposed by being the "perfect immigrant"—but also an "illegal" one. She gives herself permission to detach from her religious, traditional, family-first Filipino culture in order to excavate a legacy of violence and abuse that, unmentionable at the time, dominated her childhood and shaped her adulthood. Throughout, she incisively navigates the ambiguities of identity that immigrants constantly face.

In *The Body Papers*, Talusan uses documents—such as immigration papers, cancer test results, and legal certificates—to map an associative path to memory and the epicenters of reverberating injury and trauma. She presents the concept of "the body" as a concentric circle that expands outward: the female body, the body of the family, the body of the Philippines, the body of a writer's work.

Talusan's interconnected accounts lift the veil of protectiveness that covers many immigrants' experiences. She removes that veil with delicacy and economy, her spare writing evoking the truth without becoming a voyeur of it, pinpointing the sources of trauma without allowing her narrative to be twisted into vindictive indictment. *The Body Papers* may be Grace Talusan's debut, but it is the considered, artful work of one who has been processing these experiences with the diligence and courage of a true writer. In its message of resilience—and the salvation to be found in books—Talusan's memoir will serve as an inspiration to thousands of young immigrants who feel the weight of secrecy and silence pressed upon them.

—PRIZE JUDGES ANJALI SINGH
AND ILAN STAVANS

THE
BODY PAPERS

GRACE TALUSAN

THE
BODY PAPERS

A Memoir

RESTLESS BOOKS
BROOKLYN, NEW YORK

First Restless Books hardcover edition April 2019

Hardcover ISBN: 9781632061836
Library of Congress Control Number: 2018948395

Portions of this book have been previously published in different form
in *ArchitectureBoston*, *Boston Magazine*, *Brevity*, *The Butter*, *Creative
Nonfiction*, *Esquire Philippines*, *Image Journal*, *The Julie Mango: International
Online Journal of Creative Expressions*, *Microchondria II: 42 More Short
Short Stories Collected by Harvard Book Store*, *Orion Magazine*, *Pangyrus*,
Salamander, *Solstice: A Magazine of Diverse Voices*, and *Tufts Magazine*.

"They Don't Think Much About Us in America" and "A Way of Coming
Home" used with permission by the estate of Alfrredo Navarro Salanga.

All interior photos from the author's archive, except where otherwise specified.

Cover design by Strick & Williams

Set in Garibaldi by Tetragon, London
Printed in Canada

3 5 7 9 10 8 6 4 2

Restless Books, Inc.
232 3rd Street, Suite A101
Brooklyn, NY 11215

www.restlessbooks.org
publisher@restlessbooks.org

For mga pamangkin, *who I love like my own children*

For those who told their stories first so that I could tell mine

For Alonso, my love, my family

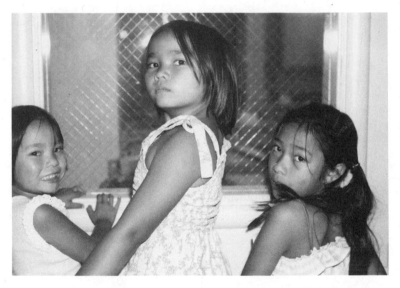

Grace age 7 (center) with sisters Ann (left) and Tessie (right).

CONTENTS

AUTHOR'S NOTE

My story is not only my story. While everyone has the right to report their own lives, I know that telling my secrets impacts other people. To preserve their privacy, I have changed the names of most living family members and friends who appear here. In some instances, I named people with a Tagalog word for our kinship tie.

This book is a memoir and is based on my memories, but I also cross-referenced documents, photographs, records, timelines, elementary school report cards, and the journals I've kept since I was a child. Still, some may dispute my recollection of events. Others may wish I had not written down such things for everyone to see.

Because I wanted to protect others from my story, I did not share or write about these memories as nonfiction for a long time. Once I became an aunt and held my niece for the first time, tiny and only days old, I realized how dangerous it was to protect the wrong people by telling only the happy stories. Lies of omission created the conditions that allowed someone more powerful than me to hurt and exploit me for most of my childhood.

At this point, I've waited long enough that many implicated in this book have died. I didn't write this book for them. I wrote it for me, and for you, the living, and for those who come after me.

THE
BODY PAPERS

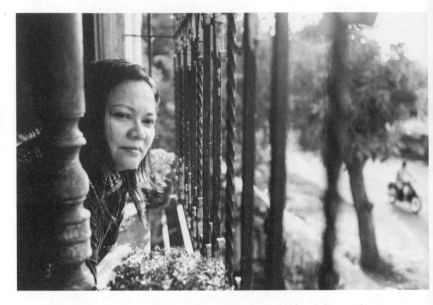

Grace leaning out of the window at her mother's family home about a three-hour drive north of Manila. The compound was commandeered in World War II by the Japanese military as a headquarters and later taken over by the U.S. Army after the Japanese withdrew. Photo: Alonso Nichols.

How to Make Yogurt in Manila

THE RECIPE FOR YOGURT can be contained in a single sentence: add a spoonful of yogurt to scalded milk and leave it alone in a warm place until it thickens.

It's a deceptively simple recipe that doesn't fully describe the process. The first time I made yogurt, I was in the closet-sized kitchen of my long-term rental in Manila. I wrapped a towel around the warm pot of heated milk as if it were a baby fresh from the bath and tucked it into the microwave oven, the door ajar so that the light bulb stayed on. I let it sleep until morning. I felt the anticipation and excitement of a childhood Christmas morning as I reached into the microwave and unwrapped the towel. The pot felt warm, but it didn't slosh. I lifted the lid and broke the white surface with my spoon. The milk had thickened into a creamy solid. At first, I was reluctant to put the warm substance into my mouth, but it was delicious. Smooth, mild, and unlike anything I'd ever tasted. It was such an unexpected marvel that I walked a spoonful to the bedroom and woke my husband Alonso from a deep sleep so that he could taste the magic too.

My beginner's luck motivates me to try for perfection again and again. I experiment with different processes, shorter and longer incubation periods, and several brands and fat contents of milk and yogurt starter. I use the milk of cows, goats, and even *carabao*, the Asian water buffalo. I play around with the consistency by straining the yogurt in cheesecloth or by adding powdered milk. Powdered milk in the Philippines is a revelation. This is not the chalk dust of my American childhood. Opposite the baby formula aisle is "adult milk," an exquisite yellowish powder that tastes like clouds and sweetness, like your mother soothing you back to sleep after a nightmare.

Eventually, I decide that carabao yogurt yields the best results. Filipino farmers depend on the carabao for growing rice and sugar; for transportation; and for milk, meat, hides, and horns. When we travel outside of the city, I always look for the hefty carabao stepping slowly through the flooded rice paddies—a beautiful brown beast amidst a landscape of palm fronds and grasses. The green looks electric after being in a city of skyscrapers, condo buildings, and malls—with its haze of gray dust covering everything and everyone. Every night in the megalopolis, I wash this dust off my skin, comb it from my hair, and blow it out my nose.

*

For the first time since I was two years old, I am living in the country where I was born. I visited the Philippines briefly with my parents a few times in my twenties and honeymooned there with my husband in my thirties, but this time I will stay here half a year, long enough for me to celebrate my forty-second birthday. We've rented a studio apartment from my cousin Jojo in BGC, Bonifacio Global City, a high-end shopping and entertainment area in Metro Manila, the capital city of the Philippines. This is the land where I began, Luzon, one of 7, 641 islands, give or take, that comprise the body of this archipelago nation. I've returned to the place where I was born because I've always had the feeling that I was missing something, like the insistent ache of a phantom limb.

*

I could not imagine what my life in the Philippines would look like, which made planning for it difficult. My husband and I prepared for the journey over many months: shopping for mosquito spray and sunscreen, subletting our apartment, settling job responsibilities, and filling out government forms. I worried about access to clean drinking water and how best to traverse Manila, famous for its gridlock. I spent hours with my sisters auditioning just the right song I could perform in case someone handed me the requisite karaoke mic at a Filipino party. I had read in an alarming article in the *New York Times* that people had been killed for sub-par renditions of Frank Sinatra's "My Way."

I had fewer immigration hurdles to navigate than my American-born colleagues on the same Fulbright fellowship trip, whose blood and stool were tested before they were granted a visa by the Philippine consulate. Unlike them, I could invoke *balikbayan* privilege as a former Filipino resident. At the travel clinic, my husband and I submitted to vaccines for rabies, hepatitis, and typhoid, and were given a yellow card certifying the ways we had protected our bodies from the threats we were about to encounter.

During the preparations, I had joined a Facebook group for foreign women living in Manila. Many of the women in the group, although not all, are the non-Filipino spouses of men who work for their home nation's consulates, global corporations, or nonprofits. As wives and mothers, they share information about the best doctors, schools, supermarkets, and other concerns. They are like me and not like me.

Upon arriving at my rental, which had not been occupied for over a year, I discovered it had been taken over by tiny ants. They traversed in orderly lines across the bathroom, kitchen, and under my bed, and when I woke up in the mornings, I swear I could feel them crawling over my scalp. When I reached the last of my drinking water, contained in an opaque blue plastic box, I was horrified to discover it thick with drowned ants. The women in the Facebook group suggest borax and solve my ant problem quickly and permanently.

Many posts in the group are devoted to the topic of household helpers: how much to pay them, how many days of vacation and sick time to give them, which ones are available for work, which ones to avoid. Help is cheap, and you don't have to be wealthy to have a household staff of drivers, housecleaners, and a nanny for each child. I often feel uneasy reading the complaints the women from Australia, Europe, and the U.S. have about their Filipino helpers, but still I post a request for a housecleaner recommendation. Someone explains that there are four kinds of people in the Philippines: A, B, C, and D. Your grade correlates with your wealth, social connections, education, and skin tone. Helpers are not generally A and B grade people, she says, and without their ma'am by their side, they could never get past the security guarding the glass doors of elite shopping malls.

The first person I hire to clean my apartment doesn't work out. She seems to scowl at me while she's mopping the floor, but I don't take it personally. She also cleans the apartment of my friend Joanne Diaz, who reports that our housecleaner complains that I shed too much hair. She seems outraged by my very existence, wanting Joanne to explain to her multiple times "what kind of a Filipino" I am.

I am the kind of Filipino whose parents left to look for a better life elsewhere. And I'm not alone. Filipinos who work overseas are top contributors to the nation's gross domestic product. As for my hair, I can understand why the woman complains about sweeping it up, strand by strand, from the floor. It could be the stress of being back in Manila after a lifetime's absence. Or maybe my body is still adjusting after losing my ovaries the previous year.

I probably should clean the apartment myself, but for the first time in my adult life, I feel I have economic power. With the U.S. dollar so strong, I have enough money to hire someone to scrub my shower and wash my clothes and drive me around so that I can focus my energy on reading and writing. I am grateful for this new luxury of time and energy. I never forget that someone else's work makes mine possible.

A couple of weeks later, I notice a popular thread in the Facebook group about making yogurt. Why would anyone bother? Our fancy supermarket, geared to foreigners, sells a variety of yogurts in the brightly lit dairy case, but the women complain that the overly sweet, watery yogurt available in Manila is many times more expensive than what they're used to paying at home, and that some local brands add chewy, gelatinous cubes for texture. One woman claims that by making her own yogurt, she was saving a thousand pesos a month on groceries, the price of a nice dinner out for four or an imported paperback.

I had never encountered such passion for yogurt, a substance I associate with the good intentions of a Monday morning. I have started many a diet at the beginning of the work week tucking a container of yogurt in my purse—and inevitably giving up on the both yogurt and the diet by lunch, when it was time to eat the watery, warm gloop.

I get why these women want their yogurt. When you can't find what you assume will always be there for you, waiting on a shelf next to the cheese, suddenly you're desperate for it. Every day in Manila, something upsets my expectations, which is a feeble way of saying what I fear makes me ungrateful, ugly, and so American: every day here, I am offended. I am appalled by the rotting inequality, greed, corruption, and lawlessness. I worry for the men working construction in the dozens of build-ings being erected in the area I'm living in, whose daily income would just about cover the cost of my morning Starbucks. On my way to get coffee one morning, I pass a commotion at the building site two blocks from my condo. A group of men had fallen from the bamboo scaffolding several stories up and two of them died. Of course, unfair labor practices exist in the U.S., but now that I'm living in this overcrowded city of 10 million, it's harder to look away from the bodies at my feet.

We feel their presence above us as we walk from our condo to a restaurant or to the gym. My friend Joanne, a poet, writes a poem called "The Ghost Workers" about these men who would not be allowed to enter the buildings they make:

> Once done, the workers who swung from one window
> to the next will be invisible to wealthy Westerners
>
> who live here. As long as the skyscrapers shine,
> as long as the rebar vanishes beneath a patina
> of glossy stone. Anyone looking for an emblem of
>
> globalization, that grandchild of empire,
> should look to those who fall to their deaths
> to strengthen its foundation.

I would much rather distract myself with dairy products. Women in the expatriate Facebook group share unexpectedly compelling recipes and processes, as well as the best places to get starter cultures and milk. They also inadvertently reveal tiny glimpses into their lives, and I like imagining their families gathered in the kitchens where they incubate their yogurt.

*

In Manila, people don't know what to make of me. I appear to be Filipino, but the way I move and speak and stand blurs easy identification. Strangers often ask me a series of questions to try and pin me down. "Where are you from?" "What is your family name?" "Do you speak our language?" Because we have so much time to kill in traffic, taxi drivers ask, over and over again, the most painful question: "How many children do you have?"

I implore the driver to let me sit in the front passenger seat because it's the only way to distract my anxious mind from panicking in the interminable traffic. The air conditioner vent blows cold air in my face and I don't feel as cramped as when I'm in the backseat. The driver begrudgingly moves his stuff to the floor and I feel I owe him a conversation. We sit so closely that sometimes our arm hairs brush against each other. Within moments, the windshield and windows obscured by laminated licenses and authorizations swinging from their hooks, driver asks if I have children. Every single time, I consider lying to shut the exchange down, but lately, I've used these moments to gauge how I'm feeling about my new reality. Should I reveal to this stranger what's been taken from my body? I practice speaking without letting my voice crack: "I don't have children." And: "I can't have a baby anymore."

The previous year, as the days ticked closer and I attended pre-op appointments for my preventive oophorectomy, I was overcome by a fog of grief and disbelief. Until the date to remove my ovaries approached on the calendar, I hadn't realized how much I wanted to spool back the days so I could get pregnant. The surgery would give birth to the post-menopausal version of me. I begrudgingly made a deal with my body: my healthy ovaries for more quality time without ovarian cancer. I wondered who I would become once I crossed the street to walk amidst the invisible, irrelevant women in our society. At middle age, would I suddenly become a crone, a virago, a hag? I had learned these words when I was fourteen, studying for the SAT, surprised at all the ways one could express contempt for women.

"I am not a mother." Without knowing a thing about me, the driver seems insulted by my answer. *Why not?* I know I'm under no obligation to explain myself, but guilt drives much of my behavior these days, and I attempt an honest answer: "My husband and I don't have enough money"—which I realize immediately is a ludicrous thing for me to say as a foreign passenger of a Filipino taxi. What else could motivate someone to spend 24-hour shifts in the most challenging traffic conditions on the planet than the faces of the loved ones they were feeding with the fares?

And then I spin more details, trying to persuade the driver that it's much more expensive in the States than they imagine. It's because my husband and I work so much, because we don't have time, because families in the U.S. can't rely on the same web of connections, because we're still paying off our student

11

loans, because it's impossible for us to own a home in Boston, on and on. As he listens to my whining, at some point, the taxi driver takes his eyes off the line dance of trucks, vans, jeepneys, SUVs, motorcycles, and pedestrians on the road ahead so he can stare hard at me and respond with some version of: *None of that has anything to do with having a child.*

And I pull out my last card: "I can't have children because of cancer." This doesn't convey the nuances of my story—the genetic tests, the trauma my body endured as a child, the heightened risk of hereditary breast and ovarian cancers, the periodic visits from depression, the agonizing decisions I've had to make about my body—but it's a reliable conversation stopper. We shift to talking about anything else, the heat, the traffic, if I happen to know anyone who is hiring a driver in the States.

*

All you need to make homemade yogurt is a heat source, a pot, milk, and a tablespoon of yogurt. You want to make sure the milk has reached a temperature high enough to kill off bacteria, but then cools off enough to keep the yogurt cultures alive—in this case *Lactobacillus bulgaricus* and *Streptococcus thermophilus*—so they can do their transformative work. You could use a food thermometer and heat the milk to 180 degrees Fahrenheit and then let it cool to 115 degrees, or you can just watch for bubbles where the milk touches the pot. Don't over-boil it. Cool the pot until you can keep your pinky in the milk for five seconds without burning yourself. Stir a tablespoon of your starter—yogurt that has live, active cultures—into the warm milk. Cover and incubate. Thermophilic yogurt incubates at around 110 degrees, so you want to keep the temperature steady for the hours that the bacteria is active and eating the sugars in the milk.

With enough practice, the yogurt-making process becomes predictable. My obsession with variables and my chemistry experiments eventually harden into certainty. I can reproduce my favorite yogurt with the same three ingredients: an ultra-high-pasteurized whole milk, a full cream powdered milk, and carabao yogurt starter. No cheesecloth straining is necessary. I eat it with cubes of yellow mangoes and a teaspoon of brown coconut sugar sprinkled on top.

I'm embarrassed by how hard I've fallen in love with yogurt making. I wonder if this is how Jesus felt turning water into wine. When visitors find themselves sick with gastrointestinal issues, I dose them with a serving of yogurt as medicine. I give them a container casually and downplay how good it is. "Try it if you feel like it, no pressure," I say, fully aware that it will blow their mind. After eating it, they call to tell me it's the best yogurt they've had in their life. They encourage me to scale up and sell it at the farmer's market. For a moment, I consider this possibility. I buy a case of glass jars in Divisoria market and sketch labels. Could I really do it? I fantasize about leaving one life for another. Is this what my parents dreamed would happen when they left the Philippines for America?

*

It isn't until my fifteen-year-old niece Naomi asks me why I am always talking about yogurt that I realize how important it has become to me. An obsession, but also a distraction. A way to avoid talking about what I encountered one morning before brunch at Purple Yam, a boutique restaurant in a historical home in Malate. The taxi dropped me off on the corner beside a blue wheelbarrow, which was full of garbage and covered with a piece of cardboard. Poverty was never far from sight in Manila. The destitute persist right outside the guarded walls of the oligarchs. The eating experience that I had prepaid for would easily feed a Filipino family for a month. As the taxi drove away, I noticed how empty the street was on a Sunday morning and my skin prickled with fear. I turned my head to the wheelbarrow and spotted the bare legs of a child sticking out from under the cardboard. My knees loosened and I grasped my friend's arm as I began to fall. I was sure that it was a child's body rotting in the heat—but then I saw the child's mother, who was also asleep just behind the wheelbarrow, on her own piece of cardboard, with two other small children and a baby beside her.

On another video call with Naomi, I talk about yogurt to avoid talking about the girls I had met at the orphanage in Marikina, girls who looked like her. I was invited to teach a writing workshop and gave the girls paper and crayons and asked them to imagine their future. "Draw what you want to be when you grow up." I expected the girls to draw what I would have as a child: astronaut, doctor, president. "Dream big," I instructed.

All of them drew pictures of fathers, mothers, and children holding hands. They dreamed of becoming daughters. A girl

I spoke with was left for dead as an infant and found under a bush covered by ants that had already started doing their work. I met another shy, slight girl, found in a cemetery, who everyone thought was thirteen, but turned out to be seventeen once her paperwork caught up with her. This girl had survived for five years among the headstones, eating the beautifully laid out oranges and pastries that mourners left as sustenance for their dead. I imagine her slipping between the iron bars of mausoleums during typhoon season to stay dry and sometimes sleeping in the cool dirt of a newly dug grave to relieve the heat. When I think of this girl living at the cemetery, I imagine her alone on the lawn above the bones, but the reality is that in Manila, some cemeteries are crowded with families who've lived among the city of the dead for generations.

I cannot describe to my niece the expression on the girl's face as the orphanage director introduced her to me, retelling her story. The orphanage had tried to find her a family to join, but now she was only a few months away from being a legal adult. She would not become somebody's daughter. Even though she probably heard the director tell her story many times, her face fell the way my knees did when I was standing beside the wheelbarrow.

"Never mind," the director said. He patted the girl on the head. "You will always have a home with us."

He turned to me. "She is training to be a caretaker for the younger children here."

Perhaps it would have been better if her paperwork had stayed lost and she'd remained a minor for a few more years—but life here is unpredictable and full of such children who cannot catch a break. The director put a baby in my arms. "Isn't she cute?" he asked. I agreed.

"Then take her to America," he said. I handed the baby back. "Joke *lang*," he said, grinning. "I'm just kidding."

*

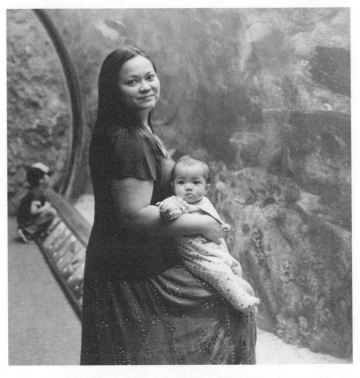

Grace holds her baby niece at the aquarium with her nephew crouching behind her. Photo: Alonso Nichols.

Since I cannot have children, I aunt. All my life, I wanted to be a mother, and once this became impossible for me, I grieved for these future unborn children that I would never know. I hid this sadness. There were several months when both of my sisters and both of my sisters-in-law were pregnant, and I did not want to spoil their joy. When I spotted a pregnant woman in public, I felt both angry and sad—angry because she reminded me of my sadness. I thought I was doing a good job of hiding my feelings until my five-year old nephew Evan asked why I only wore black. "I don't," I said, but when I looked through my closet and drawers later, I saw that almost every item of clothing I owned was black, including socks and underwear.

Aunting is sacred work. I love my dozen nieces and nephews with the fierceness and passion that I would have devoted to my own children. I am there for my nieces and nephews in the uncomplicated way that someone who is not their parent can be. I take them on excursions to museums, aquariums, malls, and historical sites. I help them with their schoolwork. I listen to their meandering stories. I advocate for their needs with their parents. I buy them as many books as they want. I try to protect them. I tell them stories about ways that people have been hurt, so that they can avoid walking behind a horse, wearing a loose robe while cooking eggs over the gas burner, stepping into a street while staring at their phone, and on and on. I know I can be overzealous with my warnings: more than once my nieces and nephews have complained that I'm scaring them.

Since Naomi was a year old, I've spent one day a week with her. When my sister Ann was pregnant, I dreamed of a little girl who would come out of the clouds to talk and play with me. I did not remember this dream until one morning at a children's museum with Naomi when she was a toddler. She burst out of the playhouse and I suddenly recognized her, that little girl from my dreams.

I talk about yogurt because I don't want Naomi to know what it means to be unlucky and unprotected. She's about the same size as the girl who lived in the cemetery, and the countless other girls I see night and day, at traffic lights, under bridges, on sidewalks, and amidst the informal settlements. I see girls who are more fortunate than those on the streets, serving as nannies and house cleaners. At least they are inside a house. If those girls were in school, they would be learning geometry and biology like my niece.

I don't want to tell my niece about the white men strolling through the malls with their Filipina girlfriends, decades apart in age. These men are suddenly peso-wealthy and far from home in Australia, Europe, and the U.S., where they would be overlooked. They strut in their sweaty tank tops full of self-importance, a young Filipina teetering in heels at their elbow. To dissipate my rage, I lie to myself that these men will buy the women's parents a house and pay tuition bills for their siblings, even their distant cousins, so that all these girls can become nurses and engineers, so that they wouldn't have to pretend affection for men like them.

I underestimate my niece. She's lived the unfairness of life.

She knows already. She lost an eye at age two. She knows our family's history with hereditary cancer and asks questions that slice through the silences and secrets we keep around trauma. And she pays attention. By ten, my niece already knew the word "rape." Uncomfortable as I was to hear this word in her girl voice come out of her girl mouth, I was relieved that she'd been warned about what can happen, about what people can do to hurt each other. As close as we are, I have not yet told her what happened to me.

Naomi understands that some people are treated as more human than others. She knows the schools—Marjory Stoneman Douglas High School, Sandy Hook Elementary School, Santa Fe High School—and she knows the names—Trayvon Martin, Michael Brown, Eric Garner, Tamir Rice, and, from the town we grew up in, DJ Henry. She fears for the men of color in her life. But of course, she doesn't think of them as "men of color." These are the men she loves: her father, brother, grandfathers, cousins, and uncles. She tells me that during an active shooter lockdown at school, if she doesn't hurry up and get into a classroom before the doors are barricaded, the teachers will not allow her inside. She decides this policy is fair—it would be her own fault for not making it into the classroom before it was locked. I turn my face away from her so she can't see my tears as I imagine her running alone through the hallways of her school, desperately trying to find an empty locker or a closet to hide in while a boy with a gun hunts.

*

Since Naomi could speak, she has always asked me to hold her tightly. I am touched by her requests for physical affection—it had never occurred to me that one could ask to be hugged and kissed and comforted. I want to show her my love, but as she passes through the ages I was when I was abused, I've become frightened of mangling a child's yearning for physical affection and the warmth and safety of love. She's old enough to know, but I still haven't been able to share what altered me. Instead of asking to be hugged, she's learned to put her hand in mine and tell me she loves me.

I've struggled with depression and the after-effects of trauma nearly all my life. The healing process has been long and complex—I've been in some form of treatment since I was sixteen. While therapy has kept me alive, sometimes I mourn the time and money I've spent. I could have paid off my student loans and bought a house, but instead every month, I pay the equivalent of rent toward my mental health: its own kind of home. It isn't productive to think about what my life would have been like without abuse and mental illness, but sometimes I see her, the woman I might have been, in my students or in women I admire. In my niece I see her future.

*

There are so many ways that life can break your heart. I don't want to burden Naomi with what makes me sad about being "home" in the Philippines. Besides, despite all the bad news, life still delights and surprises me. People come together to rescue those who need help. People still fall in love. I sometimes run into blood relatives in the city streets of Manila, something that I never experienced in America. I talk to Naomi about yogurt because I want her to believe in wonder and magic, in alchemy, in something invisible and alive that can transform liquid into solid.

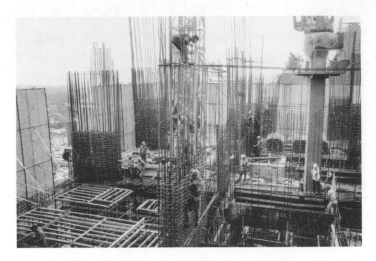

View of construction workers building Trump Tower Manila from the 33rd floor of the Gramercy Residences at Century City in Makati City. Photo: Alonso Nichols.

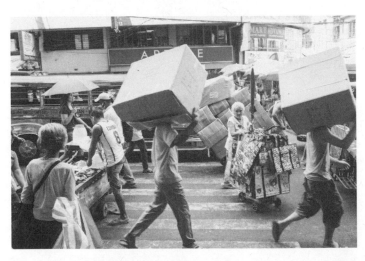

A crosswalk in the Divisoria market area in Manila. Photo: Alonso Nichols.

2

Crossing the Street

I HAVE NEVER FELT so viscerally inconsequential and expendable as when I am crossing a street in Manila.

Now that I'm living in my country of origin, I want to be a good guest. I make sure to be a model pedestrian. I always wait for the walk signal and cross inside the white lines, but I never move fast enough and wheels nip at my feet. Cars do not stop, and it is up to me to dodge them as they cross in front of me. It doesn't do any good, but I swear at drivers and yell, "I'm a person!"

In my previous family vacations in the Philippines, I never had to cross a street. My parents were overprotective, and I was always driven to the door of whatever restaurant, museum, or venue I was visiting. My skin was never exposed for long to the browning powers of the tropical sun. But now that I'm living in Manila with my husband, with the traffic and the expense of hiring a car and driver, I've decided that walking is the most efficient way to travel. But I've become fearful of crossing the street, and it becomes a source of great stress. Later, I find out that my fears are grounded. About one pedestrian is killed every other day in the city. One-quarter of those killed are children. Just outside the bubble tea place I frequent, a pregnant woman was hit while she was in the crosswalk. A speeding SUV hit another SUV that then struck the woman. A month after the accident, two hundred people paraded there to raise awareness for pedestrian safety. She led the walk in a wheelchair.

I am not prepared for this sudden intimacy with vehicles, which seem more animal than object. They are heavy-breathing creatures, their hot metal bodies close to my flesh. As a pedestrian, I am fully aware of my low position on the food chain, below black SUVs with opaque windows, motorcycles, white taxis, overloaded buses, trucks, construction vehicles, and jeepneys, long passenger vehicles whose original design came from the U.S. military after World War II. There are also trikes, motorcycles with passenger sidecars, and pedicabs, like trikes, except human-powered. People and vehicles make contact with astonishing frequency and casualness. More than once, I watch cars tap pedestrians, who then seem apologetic. My husband is hit, thankfully uninjured, by a car backing up, and yet the driver, behind dark glass, doesn't even bother to acknowledge the contact.

While living in Manila, I become afraid to cross the street, an activity I thought I had mastered as a first grader. In America, you're taught that pedestrians have the right of way, and I'm flummoxed when vehicles in the Philippines don't defer to me in the crosswalk. I constantly try to be cognizant of my position as a privileged Westerner, but I hadn't anticipated needing to check my privilege at every Manila street corner.

Instead of the leisurely thirty seconds I enjoy while crossing a Boston street, in Manila I have about five. The area I live in, BGC, advertises its friendliness to pedestrians with slogans on the backs of buses and yellow signs pointing out crosswalks. But these signs are fantasy, revealing what the city aspires to be, not what it is. Trusting that the crosswalks and signs make the streets safe for pedestrians is as naïve as believing that the skin-whitening products sold in every beauty aisle and plastered on billboards can change a Filipino's skin tone to the advertised, highly coveted, pearly hue.

*

Physically, I don't stand out from the locals, but as soon as I step into a Manila crosswalk, I distinguish myself by losing my cool: I wave my arms; I raise both hands; I shout, 'Stop!' My awkward dance in the crosswalk does nothing to stop the cars coming at me. Even the sidewalks are unsafe, blocked by utility poles, debris, construction equipment, or abandoned craters. Often, I am forced into the street. One afternoon, I exit a taxi overheating in standstill traffic, when something warm brushes against my calf. I expect to see a stray dog breathing hotly on my leg, but no, behind me on the sidewalk is a motorcycle. The driver pushes his front wheel into my leg again and jerks his helmet as if to say, *Move out of my way, lady.*

Sometimes the sidewalks are taken up by small businesses, entrepreneurs notarizing papers at desks, grinding keys, or selling snacks. Once, I pass a man standing in the middle of the sidewalk, carrying a plastic sleeve of Starbucks cups as long as his leg, mixing instant coffee and hot water from a Thermos—selling not just a drink, but also the ephemeral experience of carrying a status symbol down the street. Annoying as it is to step down into the scrum of the roadway, I admire the vendors' determination and ingenuity. They are doing what they can with what they have.

*

In some ways, living in Manila, I am a small child again. In my native tongue, I have the vocabulary of a three-year-old. I don't know how to do even simple things like make a phone call. I often offend people with my crass American manners. When responding to an invitation I know I can't accept, I decline by saying, "No, I won't be able to attend," rather than saving face by saying, "I'll try," a softer "no." If I have business with someone, I get right to it instead of making conversation about their family. I tire out the people I interview with so many questions that they stop me and say, "Nosebleed," the Filipino slang to signal they've had enough of speaking English. It's such a visceral way to describe how it feels to speak in a second language, and I feel guilty that I've caused this wound by not speaking our native tongue.

I've always wanted to know what it feels like to blend into the crowd. Growing up, I could count the other families of color in my town on one hand. Initially I sought out the few girls at school who looked like me, adoptees from Korea and China. But we had little in common. After an incident in the first grade, when a third grader danced around me making *ching-chong* sounds while pulling back the corners of his eyes, I did everything I could to be like everyone else. I practiced the Boston accent until it felt like my own. I wore green on St. Patrick's Day to be as Irish as my classmates. I prayed before sleep for God to transform me into a white girl. When I did not wake up blonde and blue-eyed, I changed my prayer: a white girl with brown hair and brown eyes would be okay. Over the years, I've developed the habit of scanning any place I enter—a classroom, a workplace, a party—searching for the faces of people who look like me. I don't expect to find them, but I still look.

Over the years I've been teaching college, a few of my students ask if I am Filipino. The Filipinos they knew from back home, they explain, were their drivers, domestic helpers, and nannies. I am often the first Filipino they've encountered at the front of a classroom. To this day, I have to remind myself that I have every right to be in spaces where everyone else is white. A few times, my students walk out of their classes to march in solidarity with nationwide protests against racism. A major concern has been the underrepresentation of Black students and faculty. They're tired of being the only ones in the room. Like me, they want to be part of the crowd.

*

On arrival in my birth country, I was fascinated by the frenzy of activity that greeted me in the airport—dazed travelers dragging heavy luggage; returning Filipino workers flush with money and gifts, known as *pasalubongs*, bought with earnings from contract work in the Middle East and Hong Kong; relatives calling out to their loved ones from van windows and the backs of pickup trucks. There was music, laughing, and the joy of reuniting with a loved one after an absence. I watched as women working as nannies greeted their own children who had grown taller than them in their absence. Men working in the oil fields or on construction sites returned with stories to tell and stories they can't. For the first time in my life, I looked like everyone else. "There sure are a lot of Filipinos here," I said to my husband. So many that I couldn't count them.

Before arriving, I tried my best to relearn Tagalog, the first language I spoke. But I can communicate only at a toddler's level, simple words such as "yes" (*o-po*) and "no" (*hindi*). The only complete sentence I can say in Tagalog is "I don't speak Tagalog." Thankfully, almost everyone I encounter in Manila speaks English, which had been introduced during the U.S. colonial period and is one of the nation's official languages. Once I open my mouth, my American accent marks my difference immediately. Almost everyone I interact with wants to chat about who I am, where I have come from, and why I am in the Philippines. So much seems possible. In Manila, I become aware of how much power and privilege I possess, something that wasn't so clear back in Boston.

Even though I am new to the city, I feel at home. Still, I am sometimes misread.

*

My best friend, Joanne, is living in Manila for a time as well, with her family. She is one the few white faces here. For the first time in our decades-long friendship, Joanne is in the minority. I wonder how she'll adjust. One afternoon, I'm with Joanne and her toddler son. I'm dressed in sweats, having just come from the gym. We enter a building, and as Joanne talks to the security guards, I wheel her son's stroller into the lobby. Suddenly, two young men brush past me, pushing me out of the way without an "excuse me" so that they can get to the elevator first. I am startled by their rudeness until I catch a glimpse of myself in the elevator's reflection. They've assumed that I am Joanne's nanny, her *yaya*, and treat me accordingly.

This, I discover, is the other side of looking like everyone else. After that, I think twice about offering to push Joanne's stroller. Even while I blend into the crowd for the first time, Joanne is experiencing the privilege of her identity as a white woman on a whole new level. Strangers comment on the beauty of her light complexion, admiring its whiteness. Joanne never opens a door for herself the entire time she's in the Philippines. When she waits in a line at the supermarket, the cashier tries to wave her to the front, encouraging her to cut ahead of Filipinos. She always refuses.

I am initially surprised, and then jealous, as I watch Joanne, technically a minority in the country, being adored and enjoying near celebrity status. And then it occurs to me that when I had been teased as a child, it may have been less about the fact that I looked different from everyone else than, quite simply, because I wasn't white. Here in my ancestral home, hundreds of years of colonialism and decades of U.S. military presence are visible everywhere, and a fascination with light skin tones is just another way that history left its mark. Many beauty products contain skin-whiteners, and I notice most local models and actors are light-skinned. I lose my temper, which is uncommon for me, in a store aisle while trying to find an antiperspirant without a skin-whitener. "Am I supposed to feel self-conscious about the darkness of my armpits?" I blurt to the sales clerk.

*

One afternoon as we speed away to the provinces from Manila, I watch as young elementary students disembark from their school bus. A pedestrian footbridge crosses the road further down, but they don't bother with it. I hold my breath as the small children run across four lanes of highway to the grassy median. A line of cars and trucks barrel down the highway oblivious. The children hold hands, their backpacks jostling behind them. That day, all of them make it across. It makes me think of my brother Jet, who was hit by a van at age seven while he was riding his bike. He hit his head and his skin scraped the tar of the road as he skidded across it. Jet spent several days in the hospital, but in the end, he was lucky and recovered. I think now what I thought then: it's not fair. The power difference between a van and a seven-year-old boy should humble any driver.

When I complain about crossing the street to Joanne, she's confused. What am I talking about? When she steps into the crosswalk, she tells me, almost every car makes a full stop. They wait until she is safely on the curb. Someone tells me that drivers are afraid of hitting foreigners, especially white ones. In all the years I've been friends with Joanne—a friendship that grew from band camp in high school, to being neighbors in our college residence hall, to living with each other post-graduation, to standing beside each other as we took our marriage vows, to unbelievably, living in the Philippines at the same time—I've rarely considered how our lives have been shaped by racial identity. Now this difference plays out in the crosswalk, powerful vehicles accelerating toward our bodies. I joke with Joanne that I needed her beside me every time I crossed a Manila street. But I am not kidding.

*

A few years ago, I was driving from campus to downtown Boston during a snowstorm. I was filling in on a conference panel for someone whose plane had not made it in time. New snow had fallen on the old, and the falling snow hushed the morning quiet. The streets were not yet plowed, so I used the tracks made by previous drivers as I came up over the hill near the gym. Not many people were outside. Halfway down the hill on the sidewalk there was a student, a young woman, bundled up in boots and a hooded parka. Her white earbuds danced like reins as she listened to music with her phone in front of her eyes. Maybe she was checking her email, or maybe video-chatting with someone. She seemed happy.

I released the gas to coast down the hill when suddenly the woman stepped into the road to cross, her back to me. She walked confidently, completely unaware of the danger hurtling toward her. If there had been no snow that day, I would have stopped hard, but there was over a foot of it in the street and I was accelerating down the hill. I braked and skidded and tried to steer out of it, but this collision was happening. My body felt electric. As my car slid at her, time slowed the way it does when you're in danger, when your life is about to change, and even though the moment was only a few seconds long, I had plenty of time to think. I worried about what part of her I would hit, if she might just break a few bones or if my car would do something worse. Maybe all the snow and her outerwear might soften the blow.

My brother Gerry, an orthopedic surgeon, told me that when a person is hit by a car, the bones can either shatter or crack, depending on how fast the car is going. The bones are relatively easy to fix, it's the damage to the soft tissues, the muscle, skin, and nerves, that's complicated. The news headlines, *Professor Runs Over Student*, flashed through my mind. I had enough time in that slowed moment to ask myself if I could survive the trauma of seriously injuring or even killing someone with my car. I didn't think I could. I blurted, "God help me" and prayed for a miracle. Everything was happening so silently and inevitably and all I could do was wait. The woman, still looking at her phone, quickened her pace.

My car stopped. I sat in the roadway, shaking. I rolled my window down to get her attention, but I had no energy, completely spent from the scare, and besides, what would I say to her? I watched her walk down the sidewalk and enter a building. She had no idea what tragedy she has just missed, and I felt both grateful and furious.

*

I walk about five miles a day. Anyone who knows Manila well can tell you that's too much. But given the options, walking is the most efficient way to traverse short distances. My friend Howie rides all over the city on his bamboo bicycle for work, but he is a master of urban cycling. Meanwhile, I appear to lack the skill to walk across a simple street.

Most people who commute on foot don't have an alternative to get to work and home. How they make a life amidst Manila's challenges—problems with traffic, air pollution, economic inequality, infrastructure, and corruption on a level I have not experienced before—floors me. For the most part, they seem to approach life contentedly. I see workers at the end of the day waiting in block-long lines to ride the jeepney or bus home. Some people report three-hour daily commutes, in each direction. And these are the Filipinos who stay. Many more work abroad for months without seeing their families. What they do out of love for each other is stunning.

Once I've been in the country a few weeks, I realize that I am the one who needs to change. If I am going to make a life here, even temporarily, I need to adjust. I am the visitor, the foreigner, the balikbayan, and I need to learn from my hosts.

I settle into a coffee shop near a crosswalk to study. I watch Filipinos cross the street. They do it calmly and gracefully, taking a few steps and then stopping in the middle of a busy intersection, where they wait patiently for cars to cross their path. They don't flinch when a car brushes past them. They don't scream or jump when a car speeds toward them. Sometimes they hold on to the person next to them and they cross together, guiding each other to stop or go, now, quickly.

They seem fully confident that together they will cross to safety.

3

My Father's Noose

WHEN MY FATHER WAS A BOY, his mother hung him.

Enter Tondo, a notorious and densely populated area of Manila, and stand in the kitchen of his childhood home. Look up. The crusty knot is still there, tied around the light fixture.

I imagine my father, Totoy, at ten. He hadn't graduated yet to long pants and shoes; his shorts and T-shirt were faded and soft from the wear of three older brothers.

Totoy had done something to make his mother Inang angrier than she'd ever been. And now, he was balanced on a stack of vegetable crates, a rope connecting his neck to the ceiling. He wore one rubber slipper—after slapping him on the ears, his mother tucked the other under the strings of her apron. If Totoy became dizzy and lost balance, or if Inang kicked the crates away, he might save himself by curling his fists and pulling on the noose as if it were the mouth on a drawstring bag. But his mother planted his palms to his hips and looked up at him. She didn't say a word, but Totoy clearly heard, *Don't try to save yourself. Don't you dare*.

Without moving from that height, he noticed his mother was balding. Her gray hair was loosely bunned, and there were triangles of white flesh between the comb tracks. Her body was thick and intimidating, fleshy rolls layered onto fat that testified to her eleven pregnancies. When angry, she made noise and broke things and stared until you looked away.

One by one, Totoy's siblings returned from school and work, stepped into the kitchen, and stepped right back out without a word.

With a pestle, she pounded garlic in the mortar bowl. She raised the butcher knife to her shoulder and chopped heads off fish. She'd fry the bodies for dinner and save the heads and tails for soup the next day.

What did Totoy think as he stood there watching his mother prepare dinner? That he'd never get to taste it? That she'd watch him suffocate as the knot tightened and then keep him there, hanging from the kitchen ceiling, a lesson for his siblings?

His brothers and sisters were hiding, staying far away from the kitchen. Even if his father could have been found—perhaps he was playing pool in a neighborhood bar or was earning money by pedaling a passenger from the market to their home in the sidecar of his pedicab—Totoy's father would not have saved him. Mother knows best. She told him, "I'm doing this because you're my son. You need to learn right from wrong."

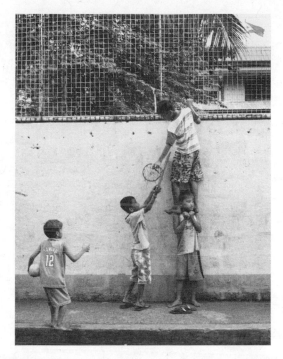

*Enterprising basketball players in Intramuros, the historic section
of Manila. As a child, Grace's father, Totoy, sometimes skipped
school to play basketball like these boys. Photo: Alonso Nichols.*

*

Totoy didn't know it yet, but he would survive. Thirteen years
later, he would have his firstborn, a daughter. But he would
never forgive his mother. Half a century later, he would not
attend her funeral. He would try to resist the urge to hit and
yell at his five children. He would do his best to protect them.
But he's his mother's son—he would fail.

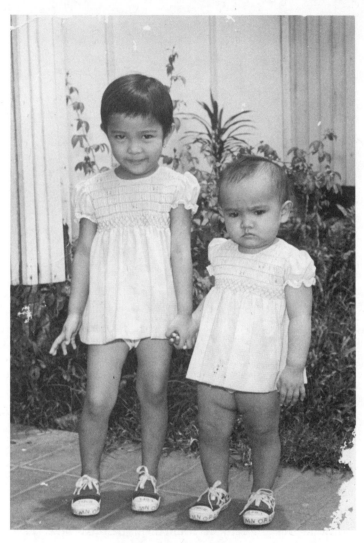

Grace at age 2 with Tessie,
her older sister, at the family compound.

4

Little Bud

BEFORE MY FAMILY EMIGRATED from Manila, I lived on a compound with blood relatives. It was our own tiny village enclosed by a wall planted with broken glass and sharp metal pieces at the top. This kept the danger out, and it also made it difficult for the teenagers and husbands to sneak out at night.

Someone always knew your business; you were never alone. Our family lived together, ate together, and prayed together. We were a large family, Catholics like the majority of the country. I was surrounded by dozens of cousins who called me by my nickname, Bubut, or Little Bud, and liked to pick me up and pinch my cheeks since I was so roly-poly. I blame my *titas*, those aunties who liked a fat child. They fed me constantly, especially *camote*, sweet potato slices fried in lard then dredged in sugar, which melted like snow on the hot coins then hardened into a shell. They liked to watch my joy as I ate.

At night, the small children glowed white with talcum powder after their baths, and the older cousins told stories until the babies' clean hair dried.

Secret histories of the family were shared: The speculation about which of the cousins were not true-blood. The story about the Muslim uncle from the south who moved to Manila as a boy when the priests offered to educate him. All he needed to do in exchange was convert to Catholicism. His family held funeral rites for him, and my uncle realized that there were ways to die before you died. Or the story of how my mother's mother, Mama Lola, was haunted by the faint sound of a crying baby, perhaps the unborn soul of her last miscarriage, and how she roamed the grounds some nights, trying to find her child.

After my mother's father Lolo died, the families on the compound feuded for months, confusing grief with anger. They stopped talking to each other, and the once vibrant compound fell quiet. On New Year's morning, Lolo's favorite holiday, the family broke their silence, all the kinfolk complaining of poor sleep. Someone had been knocking on their windows after midnight. They concluded that it was Lolo who had rapped on the glass—he knew it would force everyone back together. I grew up with the dead as present as the living. It was as if our dead family were in just the next room or traveling abroad. Sometimes they'd send you a postcard from their travels, a short and cryptic message to let you know they were thinking about you even though they were far away. Whenever we heard that a loved one had died, we asked for the time of death and recalled what we were doing when they passed. Our belief was that their soul roamed the earth for several days before moving on. Often, we would remember a strange phone call with no one on the other end, or a cryptic text message, or in my case, a single ladybug appearing on my beaker during chemistry lab in college and then flying away, leaving me with an overwhelming feeling of peace. I learned later that just before chem lab, my grandmother Inang had died.

It seemed like an idyllic place, living amongst loved ones, everyone helping each other. But soon, the membranes connecting the body of the family through daily life were ruptured.

*

My father came to the U.S. first, as a student, two years after President Marcos declared Martial Law. His plan was to study with some of the finest doctors and return to the Philippines as an American-trained eye surgeon. He was accepted to a U.S. medical residency program and anxiously awaited the paperwork from immigration. His start date at the American hospital came and went and still no visa, so he telegrammed the place, begging them to hold his spot. The hospital was well within its rights to give the residency to someone else, but they agreed to give him a few more days. If they hadn't allowed him that one grace, who knows what would have happened?

My father is an optimist. With the deadline approaching, he proceeded as if the visa were a certainty and prepared for the move. He visited his dentist, who advised him to extract all of his natural teeth except the two healthiest ones. My father didn't grow up with regular dental care or fluoride in his water.

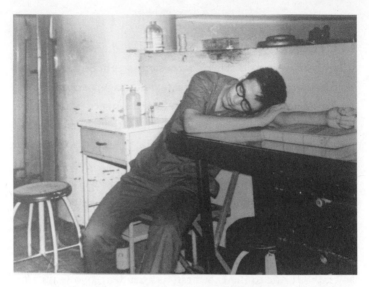

Grace's father Totoy taking a study break as a medical student.

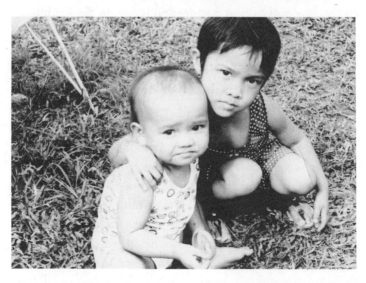

Grace before age 1 with older sister Tessie at the family compound in Manila.

"It is better to lose your teeth in the Philippines," his dentist said, "than all of your money in America."

My father feared the pain of extraction, but he dreaded the unknown expense in the States more. He opened his mouth to the dentist's pliers.

At the Chicago airport, a porter loaded his suitcase into the taxi. It was the first time my father had ever spoken to a Black man. My father tipped him a coin and the man stared at the silver in his palm before returning it. "Sir, I think you need this more than me," he said.

A few weeks into his residency, my father sent for my mother Norma, my older sister Tessie, and me. He started moonlighting as a general physician at a prison on nights and weekends. We were supposed to stay for one year only, no big deal. But this is the danger of change: you never know what else will shift.

We planned to return home to Manila with the pasalubongs that my mother had been collecting for her family: plush towels and high-thread-count sheets from the clearance rack at Filene's Basement and Jordan Marsh in downtown Boston. My father never thought he could make a life in the U.S., but he began to dream. Who could we become if we stayed?

In the meantime, my mother started working at the same hospital as my father. Although Norma had been trained as a radiologist, the researcher my father worked for hired her to work in his ophthalmology lab. Years later, after the researcher died, we found my mother's name, Norma Talusan, listed as a co-author on the papers he published from their work. She gave birth to my younger sister Ann, a natural born U.S. citizen. My father decided to study for the exam for foreign medical-school graduates. He told himself that if he didn't pass the first time, he wouldn't try again. After spending every waking minute for months studying, he passed the exam, gained his medical license, and life was suddenly full of new opportunities. My father was made full-time at his job as a prison physician, with the promise of visa sponsorship from his employers. He waited one year and then two, but they never filed the paperwork. He was too afraid to ask why.

We survived our first New England winter. We moved to the suburbs of Boston, where my parents bought a house. My father left the prison to open his medical practice. My mother birthed two more U.S. citizens, Gerry and Jet. And before we knew it, one year had turned into five, and, in a blink, seventeen years passed without us ever returning home.

*

I lost my first name, Bubut, and later, even when I could hear the love in the voice of the person who had known me as a baby, I came to hate this name. Maybe in our language, it was beautiful, but in English, it sounded like an insult. I corrected them, reminding them that I was American now and only used my American name.

My first country disappeared as a place. I never heard it mentioned in the news and not too many people in my small town had heard of the place. They knew the neighbors, China and Taiwan, where toys and electronics were made. Their fathers and uncles who had served in the military knew Subic and

Clark military bases and could say, *Mahal kita*. We were not an affectionate family during those difficult early years, so I did not know that they were parroting *I love you*, nor did I wonder who taught those men that phrase.

This is what happens when assimilation brings erasure: I lost my first language, Tagalog. My parents wanted us to embrace English only. They believed Americans would discriminate against us if they heard an accent in our voice. My parents still spoke to each other in Tagalog if they wanted to talk about us without moving out of earshot. We learned to listen closely when we heard our names popping from their otherwise indecipherable sentences. My mother told me that her parents did the same thing to her, except in Spanish, a language they continued to speak with pride, a marker of their class status and education, long after the colonizers had left.

Inside a few cells in my brain, I believe there's a part of me that still knows Tagalog. I feel pain when I attempt to speak it, as though there is something I want to say desperately that can be expressed only in my first language. But I can't access words, or that part of me that named the world first in Tagalog. When I hear strangers speaking Filipino languages, I am as drawn to them as kin.

*

We didn't return to the family compound in Manila until twenty years had passed. When we finally went back, it looked as though our house had been through an earthquake. Everything was in ruins. Even the walls had caved in, so that what was once our home had now become a small room full of junk.

My father stood in the doorway and grabbed a piece of the rubble. It was a marble nameplate that used to sit on his desk in the medical practice he worked in before having to start all over again in the U.S., retraining as a resident and then re-taking the boards.

In the Philippines, people had heard of our names. We were known. On my father's side, my uncle Dr. Tony Talusan had been a famous doctor on a long-running TV show about healthcare and the country's poor. On my mother's side, there were musicians, politicians, and businesspeople. We had a history and a context here. In America, we always had to correct people's pronunciation.

My father handed the nameplate to me and said, "I'm giving this to you so that you can always remember my name."

The marble was heavy in my hands, a miniature gravestone, and I traced the script with my finger, reading his name aloud. The afternoon light shone brightly on my father's face. His hair was starting to gray. By this time in his life, some of his friends had already died. He was trying to tell me something, but I didn't understand it at first. I wondered what kind of daughter he believed I was—one who could forget her own father's name?

*

While we lived at the family compound, my father earned extra money by making artificial eyes. I've heard stories from my cousins who watched him make these eyes while they played in the shared courtyard.

Although it was only a sideline business, my father had become known as the best maker of cheap prosthetic eyes in the city. He could make all varieties of brown eyes and took pride in the process the way someone might enjoy cooking or any activity that transforms the mundane into the sublime. First, he would press the clay-like material into the eye molds until they dried. Then, he'd paint on an iris and pupil. Next, he'd place red threads across the white to mimic veins over a sclera. He'd finally place a sheet of plastic over each eye and drop them in the boiling water to melt together.

I can see my father leaning over a metal stockpot, his shirt hanging dangerously over the orange coils of the hot-plate burner, as he checks if the water is boiling. He chews on a red thread, the same thread that he uses to create veins. What does he dream this money will buy him? He stirs the pot, taking pride in the delicacy of the process. He thought it was beautiful, how the eyes bobbed and floated and rolled over—all those eyes that couldn't see.

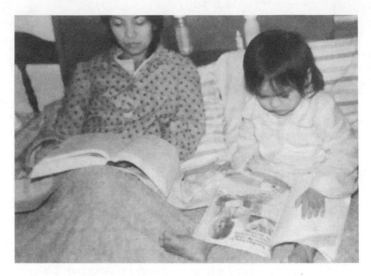

Grace age 3 with her mother Norma, who is studying to take the exam for foreign medical graduates so that she can practice medicine in the U.S. She did not end up practicing, even though she had been trained as a radiologist in the Philippines.

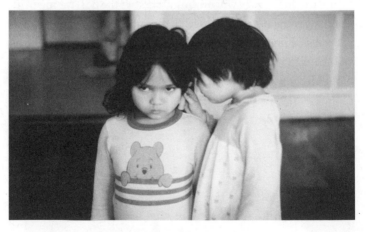

Ann telling Grace age 4 a secret in Boston.

5

My Mother's Silver Scissors

FROM CHICAGO WE MOVED to Boston and we lived in various apartments in Roslindale and Mattapan until I was in first grade. Before I understood what I was eating, my favorite meal was *lengua* in tomato sauce over a steaming mound of rice. I didn't know I was eating cow tongue, but I was five years old and liked how it tasted and felt in my mouth, soft and chewy. There were a lot of dishes that I enjoyed and only refused once I learned what it was. I loved chocolate stew with bits of chopped pork over rice until I learned its real name, *dinuguan*, and the fact that the soup was black because that's the color blood turns when it's cooked.

Before I started school, I still ate with my hands, *kamayan* style. My parents taught me to eat with a spoon and fork, but with the spoon as the primary utensil. It wasn't until I was in elementary school and eating dinner at a white American friend's house that I discovered that Americans did not set their tables with spoons unless soup was being served. I learned to eat like them by observing my friend's father stab morsels with his fork and sometimes push bites onto the fork with his knife. I ate the skin of a baked potato for the first time at my friend Kelly's house and brought this knowledge home, shocking my family by ingesting what they considered to be garbage. In elementary school, I started to refuse the spoon and showed off how I could eat with just a fork. It was more practical to eat rice with a spoon, but my parents picked their battles with us. My mother continued to set out spoons and forks and quietly collected the clean spoon from my placemat every night and returned it to its place in the drawer.

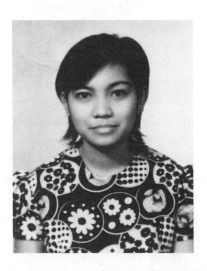

Grace's mother Norma before she left the Philippines.

As I became friends with more Americans and ate meals at their homes, I started to feel ashamed about the things we ate in our Filipino household. I no longer enjoyed my favorite Filipino foods and started to think of them that way—as foreign—whereas before they had just been food, with no ethnic preface. My older sister Tessie told me that dinuguan was made of blood and pig organs and that lengua in tomato sauce was cow tongue. I reacted the way I thought my white American friends would. "That's disgusting," I said. "Gross."

I asked my parents if it was true, that the food that I had loved and had sustained me this far in life was tainted. The next time my mother served dinuguan or lengua in tomato sauce, my mouth watered for it, but I didn't touch it, imagining what my friends would say if they knew what I ate. "Aren't you going to eat?" my father asked me.

I stared at the tongues swimming in red sauce and shook my head. I wanted to talk fresh the way my friends did to their parents and challenge them, "How can you eat a tongue with your tongue?" But I stayed quiet and ate a scoop of rice the way I saw my friend Kelly eat rice at home, with butter and salt. I remember being surprised at how quickly I became hungry again so soon after dinner.

To this day, at home, I prefer to eat kamayan style. It's the best way to separate meat from bone and fish from spine. The fish we ate at home when I was growing up had a head and tail. Sometimes I inadvertently swallowed fish spines and I'd panic at the pins in my throat, standing up from the table and mouthing, "Spines."

My parents weren't worried. "Swallow a mound of rice whole without chewing," my father told me.

"Find a cat," my mother would say. "Pick it up and let it scratch at your throat." I looked at her like she was crazy. "In the Philippines, they say that if you have fish spines stuck in your throat, you should let a cat scratch your neck and the spines will come out." She laughed. "It doesn't make sense now that I think about it."

I had only stayed for two years in the Philippines, but in my family home I still lived there. Every time I left the house, I crossed a border. As much as I had to adjust to cultural differences, I wondered what that meant for my parents, raising children in America, these strange and ungrateful foreigners.

Once we moved to the suburbs, my mother was more relaxed, but for the first several years after we arrived in the U.S., she was a different woman. I can see now that it must have been incredibly difficult and lonely for her to leave everyone and everything she loved and needed and to find herself in a tiny apartment with three small children and no one to help her. The person she is today would never dream of treating children the way that younger version of her treated my sister and me. She was young and scared and new to mothering us full time. Once she learned that you were not supposed to hit small children with slippers and leather belts and rolled-up magazines, she stopped. She was only repeating what had been done to her.

To save money, she cut our hair at home. Some of my earliest memories of my mother is sitting in a chair with a plastic poncho around me while she cut my hair. I loved having all of her attention on me for once. She was focused on making me beautiful. She told me to sit still. I saw the flash of the gleaming scissors and listened to the satisfying sound of my bangs being cut, a kind of chewing sound. Sometimes my hair fell between the poncho and my neck and it tickled. I squirmed. My mother said, "Sit still." I shuddered when the cold blade of the scissors touched the back of my neck. "It tickles," I said. "If you don't sit still, I'm going to cut off your ears," she said. I wondered if my skin would make the same sound as a sheet of red construction paper when it was cut in half.

I was terrified of my mother's silver scissors. When I made too much noise or screamed in the apartment when the baby was finally sleeping, my mother whisper-screamed for me to be quiet. "Do you want me to cut your tongue out?" she asked with all seriousness.

"If you cut out my tongue, how would I talk?" I asked. "Can you sew my tongue back on after you take it off?"

"You ask too many questions for your own good," she said.

I remembered this threat in college when I read Ovid's *Metamorphoses*. After Philomela is raped in the woods, her rapist cuts her tongue out so that she can't talk about what he did to her. She weaves a tapestry that tells the story of her rape, setting in motion a revenge which results in the rapist, unknowingly, eating his young son. That is how dangerous a story is. My mother, now in her seventies, returned from a dental appointment recently and reported that she had a frenectomy. Her dentist snipped the band of tissue under her tongue. All this time she had been "tongue tied." One cut freed her tongue.

I have noticed that in her later years, my mother has become more outspoken, more vocal about her opinions and political beliefs, which are completely different from those she held when she first arrived in America.

*

I was a child of four or five when I finally put the scissors in my mouth. I needed to know how it would feel. I needed to face the thing I was most afraid of. I closed the pointed blade against my tongue, tasting the metal and then blood. I jumped from the sharp and sudden pain. I dropped the scissors. I had just nicked myself, barely anything. A bad word that was incredibly satisfying to say slipped out of my mouth. Remembering that dirty words made us dirty, I preemptively washed my own mouth out with the bathroom bar soap and promised to try harder to be a good and quiet girl.

I wanted to teach my tongue to behave. I taught myself how to tamp down outbursts. When I felt angry at my sisters, I stopped saying the first thing that came to my lips, "I hate you," or "I'm so mad." I stopped laughing loudly, uncontrollably, which I learned looked ugly coming from a girl. As I became quieter and quieter, people—parents and teachers alike—seemed to appreciate me more. I wanted to be a good girl. I would blow sour bubbles from the soap and gargle with water until my mouth was clean. Better soap in my mouth than no more tongue to taste the world and speak about it.

Looking back, I know my mother wasn't serious. She was just repeating a threat that someone had leveled at her when she was a child. But I was a small girl with a big imagination. I did not know the boundaries of an empty threat, of what one body could do to another's. When my mother turned into a witch with the silver scissors and threatened to cut off my ears and tongue, I believed her. I became the girl in the fairy tale who the witch hated and wanted to destroy. I became a girl afraid of being cut like scrap paper.

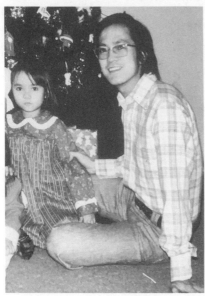

Grace age 5 with her father at Christmas in Boston.

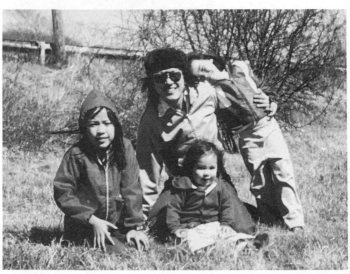

Grace age 4 with her father and sisters, Tessie and Ann.

6

Arm Wrestling with My Father

I NOTICED THAT MY PARENTS were different from other parents. At the time, I attributed it to us being Filipino, but I realize now that they were undergoing a profound change as they settled into our American life. I thought I had grown too old to be hugged, cuddled, and kissed by them, but I think they were overwhelmed and didn't have the capacity. Now that they are grandparents, they're devoted to their grandchildren and shower them with love. I'm jealous of the grandparents that my nieces and nephews have. I would have wanted them for my own.

But when they were my parents, they did not have much physical touch and affection to give. As children, we knew to greet older relatives with quick pecks on the cheek or to lift their hand to our forehead in *mano po*, a gesture of respect. I don't remember hugging my parents or exchanging "I love you"s with them until later in life.

As my parents became more American, they seemed to become more like my white American friends' parents, and were more physically affectionate with my younger siblings than with my older sister Tessie and me. Like our suburban neighbors, my parents became huge sports fans and threw Super Bowl parties where my mother served Filipino foods alongside the Super Bowl dishes she found on the packaging of processed cheese and sausages. The parents of my early childhood in Boston disappeared and new parents, unrecognizable to me, took their place in the suburbs.

My father found the neighborhood we settled in by asking around at work which town had the best public schools. We moved into a split-level ranch on an acre in a suburb south of Boston. Three bedrooms and two bathrooms, the perfect size for my family. Across one entire wall in the living room hung a mirror streaked with what it would look like if birds pooped gold. After living in apartments with wood floors, the yellow shag carpet was soft and luxurious; my feet sank until the plush threads covered my ankles. "I could sleep here," I announced, stretching out. A day or two after we moved in, I was crawling on the wall-to-wall with one of my brothers and felt a sharp pain on my right leg. I was shocked to see a sewing needle sticking out of my knee. What if the last family hid needles all over this carpet? I became afraid of walking on the yellow shag after that, unsure where injury might find me.

On the first morning after we moved from the city to the big house in the suburbs on an acre of land, I awoke to a bird chirping so loudly and clearly that I thought it was in my bedroom. It sang, "Bob, Bob, Bob White." It sang this over and over again and I listened with my eyes closed until I could not stand the sound. Who was Bob White? And why was this bird looking for him? I ran to my window where my bedroom faced the backyard. There was no bird that I could see on our swing set or the twin rocks jutting out of the grass or the leafy tree. I stared into the woods along our back fence. I could not believe all this grass was ours. I felt we had moved to a magical place like in the animated Disney movies where the flora and fauna started singing when the heroine walked past them.

*

Our house was American on the outside, but Filipino on the inside. We left our shoes at the door and wore slippers inside the house. We had a *tabo*, a small plastic container by the toilet for washing up. We had an electric rice cooker on the kitchen counter that was never empty of rice, and hanging on the dining room wall, a giant wooden spoon and fork set next to a framed velvet rendition of Da Vinci's "Last Supper." We had an altar with statues of the Santo Nino, an image of Christ as a child, and the Blessed Virgin Mary, and we would kneel together as a family in front of it to pray the rosary, especially when a relative died. We would pray a novena, nine nights straight, for the soul of a recently departed loved one. My favorite line of the prayers was when we said the name of our dead aloud and asked that God would "let perpetual light shine upon" them. I learned later that our Americans friends who came over were freaked out by all the faces of Jesus and the saints looking at them from our walls.

My brothers Gerry and Jet were conceived and born in those first years in the house, a golden, hopeful time in my parents' lives, when they worked together to establish my father's ophthalmology practice. There was more than enough room for our growing family, and relatives from the Philippines would stay with us for months.

*

For a time before I reached puberty, my father would pop his elbow onto any flat surface—the counter in the galley kitchen that my mother resented cooking in, the rickety card table piled with white and yellow mahjong tiles, or the wooden church pew before Sunday Mass—and call for me.

No one else called me "Gracie."

We clasped hands and he counted down from three. He didn't go easy on me. For the moments we were locked together, my world was my arm. Nothing mattered more than pushing his knuckles to the counter: I wanted to win. I remember telling my father about a woman I saw on TV who was so strong, she arm-wrestled against men and won.

I surprised my father by being pretty good at arm wrestling. "You're strong, Gracie," he said.

Perhaps not TV strong, but good enough to beat him occasionally. I liked having something to do with my father. He wasn't like my friends' dads, who asked them their opinions about current events. My father was a man of few words and expected fewer from me. I don't remember him telling me that he was proud of me until I was nearly an adult. By then, he had been in America long enough to adopt the excesses of its syntax.

*

My father is not a big reader, but through books, he learned how to fix his car, play tennis, and win at blackjack. Books were valuable only if they were useful. If he saw me relaxing on the couch reading a novel or a memoir, he would ask me to help him with chores since I wasn't doing anything important. Now, my father goes online if he needs to fix something broken. But when I was a girl, he found bargain "how to" books and coached me to ice-skate, swim, and high-dive, although he couldn't do any of those activities himself. He learned how to condition leather mitts until they were as soft as pillows and how to throw overhand and underhand. As we stood at opposite ends of our backyard, my father encouraged me to throw hard like a boy, both baseballs and footballs. We played one-on-one under the regulation net in the driveway and he ran me through drills: layups from the right of the basket and then the left, how to push and jostle and elbow without fouling. The only sport that I took to was soccer, and he showed up to almost every one of my games, shouting "Gracie!" from the sidelines. Above the din of the field, my ears always picked out his voice.

During those years, I played soccer most days of the week with girls whose legs were thick and heavy with muscles. We stretched and sprinted and kicked hard. We wanted to be powerful enough to kick the ball from the corner to the net. We wanted to throw the ball all the way up the sidelines.

Sometimes during a soccer game, we would be so angry that we'd growl. We wanted to win so badly that we could taste it, and when we lost, we'd spit on our hands and clap the disappointment onto the other team's palms.

*

It was my father's evening habit, after I brushed my teeth, to call me to his lap, and when I did not fit anymore, I'd sit between his legs. I didn't mind. I liked his attention and his warm fingers on my face. With his thumb and forefinger, he pinched the bridge of my nose and massaged the cartilage, coaxing it to rise from my face. He said it was for my own good; in this country, no one appreciated the beauty of a flat nose. I often pretended to be deeply asleep at the end of long drives so that my father would carry me from the car to my bed. Like I was Aladdin and my father was my magic carpet. As he flew me through the sky, my father would sing a tune that belonged to me only, a song he sang to me when I was still in my mother's womb and what I hope to hear as I die, "Sleep, my baby, sleep."

Until I was in the first grade, my father would hold my hand to cross the street so that I wouldn't get lost in a crowd. I liked holding hands with him, but like riding in a stroller and sucking from a bottle, these were eventually phased out. At some point, during the year that I turned eleven, we stopped arm wrestling. I don't remember if it was his idea or mine to stop. But it was the last time we held hands.

*

The day that I got my first period, after hearing the news from my mother, my father stood in the doorway behind me silently. I was playing video games. I sensed him there and fidgeted, still not used to the bulk in my panties and the sensation of the flow. I could tell he was trying to find the right thing to say. "I heard from your mother," he said. "You are a woman now."

I didn't know what that meant. I felt the same as before except for some muscle cramping and heightened irritation. I rolled my eyes and said, "Thanks," wishing he'd go away.

Back then I had no idea what it meant to become a woman, but I learned there were rules once you crossed the border from girlhood: No more drinking soda from the bottle; no more eating a banana upright from the peel; sit with your knees pressed together.

And what did being a woman mean after all? As a middle-aged woman, I still have moments when I feel eleven.

*

Years after the fact, my mother told me about a workshop on parenting teenagers they had both taken at our church. This was the church we belonged to since moving to the suburbs, and where we attended weekly Sunday Mass and fulfilled Holy Days of Obligation. We had our choice of two Catholic churches in town, but my parents chose this one because the Italian American pastor's last name, Phillipino, was a homophone for Filipino—a good omen. My brothers were baptized in that church and we continued with the next three of the seven Sacraments of Catholic life: Eucharist, reconciliation, and confirmation. We participated in the life of the Church by playing in the basketball league and joining the youth program where we went to dances, ski trips, and were encouraged to say no to drugs and sex. During high school, we volunteered to teach catechism at Sunday school for a new batch of Catholics. We lived in a small town, and our fellow parishioners were also our classmates, school teachers, sports coaches, accountants. My father was their eye doctor. We felt we belonged.

At this parenting workshop, my father stood to ask a question. I can see him standing amidst all the white parishioners, having to repeat himself since they couldn't understand his accent. He was hoping the workshop leaders could tell him if it was okay to embrace his daughters once they started developing breasts. What was the rule? My mother was mortified and pulled him to sit down. It occurs to me now that maybe he was scared of us, his little girls transforming into these strange, foreign creatures, these American women, before his eyes.

7

Deportable Alien

TO CELEBRATE HAVING PASSED the boards for foreign medical graduates, my father bought a new Chevy Caprice station wagon, turtle green with matching interior. The flatbed in the back folded into a bench seat that faced the rear. In the summers, we rode the highways of America in our green station wagon. I would perch on the armrest between my parents' seats while my father asked me to read the highway signs. My parents avoided spending money on fast food—instead, my mother brought freshly cooked rice and chicken adobo. I was embarrassed as I watched other families eat peanut butter and jelly sandwiches and potato chips at rest stop picnic tables.

We visited the nation's monuments and national parks, but my father's true interest was finding out how things were made. He loved a factory tour. There was no entrance fee, and you often walked away with a free sample. We watched cereal get made

RECORD OF DEPORTABLE ALIEN (See A.M. — 2790.31-.34 for Instructions)

Family Name (Capital Letters)	Given Name	Middle Name
TALUSAN	Grace	Accla

Country of Citizenship: Philippines
Passport Number and Country of Issue: 262312 Philippine
File Number: 24576659

U.S. Address — (Residence) (Number) (Street) (City) (State) (Zip Code)

07/31/74 SFR J-2 — Tokyo

Number, Street, City, Province (State) and Country of Permanent Residence
71 Drexel Tech. Univ. Hills Cal City, Phil

Date of Action: 8/11/81
Location Code: DOO

City, Province (State) and Country of Birth
Manila, Philippines

Form (Type & No.): I-94
☐ Lifted ☐ Not Lifted

Visa Issued At — NIV No. 000146
Social Security Account Name: n/a

Date Visa Issued: July 5, 1974
Social Security No.: n/a
Send C.O. Rec. Check: 50

Immigration Record: admitted until Dec 31, 1978
Criminal Record: n/a

Name, Address, and Nationality of Spouse (Maiden Name, if appropriate): n/a

Sex: 7

Marital Status: ☐ Single ☐ Married ☐ Separated ☐ Widowed ☐ Divorced

Method of disposition/Apprehension: 8042
(At/Near)   Date:

Length of Time Illegally in U.S.: Over 1 year

Possession ☐ None Claimed ☐ See Form I-43   ☐ Yes ☐ No   ☐ Not Listed ☐ Listed, Code _____   SEM1B

Name and Address of (Last) (Current) U.S. Employer: n/a
Type of Employment:
Salary: ____ From: ____ To: ____

Narrative (Outline particulars under which alien located/apprehended. Include details, not shown above, re time, place, manner of last entry, and elements which establish administrative and/or criminal violation. Indicate means and route of travel to interior.) Alien has been advised of communication privileges pursuant to 8 CFR 242.2(e).
Initial ____ Date ____

Subject is a 9 nine yrs old child.
Alienage and Dep ☐ability established.
Departure to coincide with parents

Re: Dep. to coincide w/parents

DISTRIBUTION
1 file
1 by

Form 1-213 (Rev. 4-16-79)Y UNITED STATES DEPARTMENT OF JUSTICE Immigration at the Kellogg's factory in Michigan—the air was perfumed with hot corn syrup, and I suddenly became ravenous, wanting to reach my hands into the scalding vats and stuff myself. We visited the Chevy assembly plant in Delaware, and at the U.S. Mint, we saw money being printed and fantasized about what we could do if all that money was ours. In Richmond, Virginia, we watched tobacco become cigarettes: beautiful white paper cylinders packed gently into boxes. Everyone in the family, including us kids, walked away from that tour with a carton of cigarettes.

My parents didn't like to stop often—a waste of time—even on very long car rides. They taught us to deny our bodies. My mother fashioned a car toilet out of my younger siblings' training potty to avoid bathroom stops. When it came time for her to take over driving, they danced a complicated ballet of switching drivers without ever braking: my father kept his foot on the gas and started to edge his body over to the passenger side while my mother held on to the steering wheel and kept the top of her body trained forward. When they successfully completed the maneuver, all five of us kids would cheer and clap.

When my mother wasn't driving, she was holding one of the babies in her lap in the front passenger seat. This was back when you didn't wear seatbelts or strap children into car seats. If you needed to throw something away, you rolled down your window and forgot about it. We went along with the ambitious itineraries my father put together from his AAA tour books. He believed in quantity over quality. We went along with his relentless appetite for tourist destinations without complaint until a trip to the Grand Canyon. After hours of driving, we had been freed from the hot car and were in awe at the natural wonder, none of us speaking as we stood against the guard rails. My father surveyed the expanse for about five minutes, clapped his hands, and exclaimed, "Ready to go?"

*

One trip we set off in the green station wagon to visit my father's relatives in Canada. The border agent studied our Filipino passports and our U.S. visas, which were about to expire. He saw our family's luggage and assumed we were fleeing to Canada, so he sent us away. I had never seen my parents so intimidated. Back then, anytime we encountered men in uniform—immigration officials, the DMV, traffic cops, even postal workers—my parents transformed into meek people who didn't ask questions and did what they were told.

My parents said nothing about it at the time, but when my father's student visa expired, we became what today would be called "undocumented." There was plenty of documentation that we existed—my father had bought a house, started his own business, and paid taxes. But despite that and the immigration lawyer our father hired, our paperwork took many years to process, and my parents, my older sister, and I were soon out of status, in administrative violation of the nation's immigration laws. We were advised not to leave the country if we wanted to be allowed back in.

In the Filipino community there's a term called TNT, short for *tago ng tago*. It's a Tagalog term translated literally as "hiding and hiding"—from immigration. My father tells me today that he was not scared of deportation, even though he would have lost his business, his home, and our education. Our lives would have been diverted from their paths, perhaps permanently. My mother adds that we weren't actually hiding because "immigration knew where to find us."

I was a teenager when my parents told me why I couldn't visit my cousins in Canada during the summer, or study abroad, or vacation in the Caribbean. The realization hit me: I was an illegal alien. I had heard what people said about "illegals," and how they blamed us for society's problems. My younger siblings, who had been born here, had a right to be in the country, but I didn't. The future suddenly went dark. My older sister Tessie and I could be deported to the Philippines, a place I barely remembered. I couldn't fathom starting over in a foreign nation, even though I knew that's exactly what my parents had done when they came to America.

My parents hid our immigration troubles from us until they had to tell my sister Tessie and me why we were being taken out of school for medical exams and blood tests, fingerprinting, background checks, and interviews. Our parents wanted to spare us the worry, but once I was so physically involved with immigration, I realized how precarious our status was. The whole time, I was terrified. I had never thought about how meaningful U.S. citizenship was until I was told I didn't have it. With a shuffle of papers, life as I knew it could be lost. I am still astounded by how meaningful these papers are, how they are pasted onto our bodies and determine where and how we can move through the world.

Grace age 6, in her cancelled Philippine passport.

*

Years later, after we had become U.S. citizens, my father gave me a folder with "Grace Amnesty" scrawled across it in blue pen. It was full of papers verifying that I had been living continuously in the U.S., including a letter from my church priest testifying to my good qualities. There was also a memo from the Department of Justice's Immigration and Naturalization Service asking me to voluntarily return to my country of origin with my parents.

The documents tell their own story. I entered the U.S. on the last day of July in 1974 through San Francisco. Pasted in my Philippine passport is a J-2 visa, which I was granted as a dependent of my father, who then had a student-exchange visa.

April 16, 1987

Department of Immigration and Naturalization Service
Department of Justice

To Whom It May Concern:

I have known Grace Acela Talusan since 1979. In my experience she is an

excellent student and like her sister has much musical talent. She is a

credit to her family and I am happy to give her my highest character reference.

Sincerely yours,

Rev. Lucio B. Phillipino

Reverend Lucio B. Phillipino, Pastor
Immaculate Conception Church

Letter from Grace's parish priest in support of her remaining in the U.S.

Our authorization to stay in the U.S. expired in 1978, though my father had been promised a new visa by his employer. (He worked as a physician at the local prison, where he examined alcoholics brought in from the street by the police to "dry out" overnight and tended to the wounds of those physically assaulted while in custody. One man had swallowed razor blades to get a hospital break away from the prison.)

In 1981, there is paperwork related to deportation, but then in 1988, there is a waiver granted for the foreign-residence requirement of the Immigration and Nationality Act. President Reagan's 1986 Immigration Reform and Control Act had given us a pathway, along with 2.9 million other people. At sixteen, I got my driver's license as soon as I was eligible, and I used this to hide the other card I was supposed to carry on my person at all times: my temporary resident alien card. I was mortified by it and didn't tell my friends that I was a green-card holder. I was afraid they would make fun of me for being an illegal alien. In 1995, I was sworn in as a U.S. citizen and my college friends threw me a party. I blew out candles on an American flag cake striped in red strawberries, white cream, and blueberries. For the first time in years, I felt safe.

Under Reagan, the government did not force us to return to the Philippines before proceeding on the pathway to U.S. citizenship. I think about this now, while families are being separated at the southern border, while thousands of the most vulnerable people are subject to deportation, while thousands march in protest. Is this the same government that decades ago kept my family together? Soon after Trump's inauguration and the first

Muslim travel ban, even though I had lived in America since I was two years old, I felt the tectonic plates of identity shift. I started carrying my U.S. passport with me whenever I left the house. I was not really welcome in America. At a moment's notice, I might be forced to prove that I had the right to walk these streets and teach in my classroom.

Curious about what I might find, I submitted a FOIA request. Six months later, the government sent back almost a hundred pages of immigration-related documents with my name on them. In the summary letter, I was informed that one and half pages were withheld by U.S. Citizenship and Immigration Services along with an additional eight pages withheld by U.S. Immigration and Customs Enforcement (ICE). I read that the withheld material might contain information related to the enforcement of criminal laws and the protection of law enforcement processes. The dozens of pages I had in hand seemed weightless compared to the heavy burden those missing pages placed on my mind.

When I finally received some of those redacted pages, "child" was written boldly over the parts that were not covered up. I asked my high school friend, Jeffrey Rubin, now an immigration lawyer in Boston, what they were. Jeff explained that the documents were planning paperwork and detailed how they would have gone about arresting my family for overstaying our visas. I showed my father the papers and waited for his reaction. He said, "Those aren't a big deal." I returned to Jeff and asked again what these papers meant. Jeff responded, "You were told to leave the U.S. This is heartless and exactly what they're doing to many, many people right now. They are saying, 'Get lost, you are expelled.'"

Perhaps my father's way of approaching the world, a "no worries," cavalier attitude, is the better way to be. I am careful; I worry; I research; I go over everything before I act, from making hotel and restaurant reservations to making medical decisions. I am a cautious person who does not get very much done. Perhaps my father's nature is what drove him to emigrate. He is that special kind of person who would leave everything he knew to brave the unknown with the certainty that he was moving toward a better life. My father believes everything will work out. And after all, didn't it?

*

We never had an accident in the green station wagon, but we had a few near misses. We almost had a head-on collision with a long-haul truck, a memory that is only light and sound, my parents screaming, the truck's throbbing horn, lights flooding our car like a lightning storm, illuminating our terrified faces. My father swerved and the truck flew past us like a hot, belching dragon. The other near accident happened during an ice storm in the middle of the night on a deserted highway. Us kids were sleeping untethered on the seat that folded into a flatbed when the car spun on black ice. My mother did not know to steer into the skid; this was it, she thought, our luck had run out. She turned from the driver's seat to look at her children, certain she was about to watch us fly through the window glass onto the highway, but instead there was Lolo, her dead father, hovering over her sleeping babies, his ethereal body a blanket that held them in place.

My father continued to drive the green station wagon even after he was established as a surgeon and was parking in the doctors' lot amidst luxury Mercedes, BMWs, and Audis. It held so much value for us, even if others couldn't see its potential. Finally, after fifteen years, it became time to get rid of the beloved car. He parked it on our front lawn with a cardboard "For Sale" sign. Each week, he discounted the price until eventually, he had to pay a man $200 to tow it away. The car was hitched up, and at first the end dragged on the tar, sparking orange. As the tow truck eased its way out of our long driveway, I was surprised to see my father step into the middle of the street, where he stood quietly on the yellow median until our green station wagon disappeared from sight.

8

The Gentle Tasaday

ONE DAY IN OUR FOURTH-GRADE geography unit, my teacher announced that the next country we would study would be the Philippines.

I raised my hand and waved it back and forth. "My parents are from there!" So was I, but back then, I didn't think of myself as being anything other than American.

My teacher was surprised; she thought we were Chinese. She invited my father to come and talk to the class about the Philippines.

I was queasy with excitement as I watched him spread decorations from our walls onto two desks pushed together: *Weapons of Moroland*, a black plaque of tiny metal swords from Mindanao. A lamp of round flat shells strung together. His fanciest *barong* Tagalog shirt, the one woven from *piña* cloth. It may have been the same one he wore when he married my mother. He almost included in the display a carved wooden figurine of a man sitting in a barrel. When you lifted the barrel off the man, he was naked and, boing, a stick as long as one of his legs popped straight out from the center of his body. I begged him to leave Barrel Man at home. My classmates clapped for my father, and my teacher was so impressed with the authentic Philippine artifacts that she asked him to leave the display up until our country study was over.

The next week during social studies, my teacher said, "Today we will learn about the Tasaday people. Has anyone heard of the Tasaday?" She stared right at me.

I shook my head. She went on and described a lost tribe recently discovered in the Philippine jungle. The story was that they had been untouched by modern life since the Stone Age. They were a window to humanity's early days.

"Are you sure you didn't know about the Tasaday in the Philippines?" she asked me.

I had never heard of them from my parents or anyone else, but the teacher had proof, a filmstrip. As my teacher threaded the canister of film into the projector, a boy tapped me on the back. "Do you want to see a filmstrip?" he asked.

My friend whispered loudly, "Don't answer him."

Flattered by his attention, I nodded. The boy cupped his hand around his eye as if it was a camera lens and moved his other hand in a circle next to his ear. "Good," he said. "I'll film and you can strip."

Everyone laughed and I did not know where to set my gaze. Were they picturing me taking off my clothes?

The teacher asked someone to get the lights. She explained that even though the Tasaday were backward and lived in caves, they were a noble and peaceful people, whose vocabulary had no words for "war" or "enemy."

I had no idea what the Philippines looked like. We didn't bring family photo albums with us to America, and I'd never seen anything about the Philippines depicted on the news or movies. The images on the filmstrip made me sink into my seat. The boys whooped at glimpses of breasts and bare thighs. They reacted the same way when issues of *National Geographic* with topless brown skinned women were passed around. I covered my face with my hands so no one could see my reaction. There was an old man with long earlobes and he perched like a seabird, his arms hugging his thin brown legs like wet wings. Another man with curly hair crouched near a cooking fire, his butt parted with a thick vine and a leaf wrapped around his crotch like a package. The image reminded me of one of my favorite snacks, rice and coconut milk steamed in a banana leaf, and I shivered, imagining what it would be like to open up the packet to find this man's genitals in it. A woman held a baby to her long, flat breasts, the reddish nipples pointing away from each other like lazy eyes. She stared into the camera, waiting for something. She looked at me as if to say, "You are a Tasaday, too." I expected to see this same stare from my classmates. I was used to this feeling, all eyes on the different one, the foreign other, and I hated it.

There was Lobo, a child with shoulder-length curly hair. My classmates argued over the child's gender. Boys didn't have hair like that. Someone pointed to me and said, "There's your future husband." I was mute with shame.

Another image showed a banana leaf piled high with dead frogs, tadpoles, newts, and lizards. The Tasaday squatted naked on the cave floor. Some people were sitting on large rocks, their skin dusty with ash, drying in the sun like the lizards they ate. The class came to life with noises of disgust. "They're going to eat that? That's their food?" My classmates teased me, wondering if the sandwich meat between my Wonder bread was made of reptiles.

At the time, I knew no more about the Philippines than my classmates, so I could not tell them that the Tasaday were considered a hoax. Manuel Elizalde Jr, an amateur anthropologist, introduced the group to the world, allegedly promising money to those needy folks in exchange for this performance of primitivism. And he was right. It was what people wanted to see. Briefly, the world's attention suddenly focused on the Philippines, and here I was in an American fourth-grade classroom, seeing the first images of my home country I'd been exposed to since we emigrated.

I was relieved when our study of the Philippines ended and I could dismantle the display of our family's decorations. As I loaded the things into my bag, I noticed that some of the metal blades were missing from the black plaque and some *capiz* shells from the hanging lamp were cracked. As I folded my father's barong, I noticed the shirt was stamped by multiple shoe treads. The barong must have slid from the desk to the floor. I brushed the delicate beige cloth, stiff like paper, but couldn't erase the shoe prints from its back.

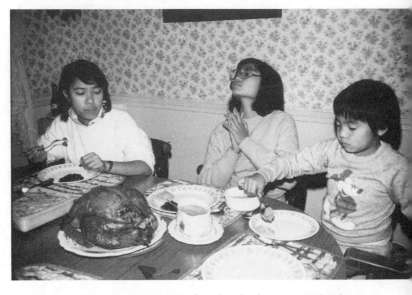

Grace (center) prays before the Thanksgiving meal with her older sister Tessie and younger brother Gerry.

9

They Don't Think Much About Us in America

by Alfrredo Navarro Salanga

Q. *Do you feel you are free to express your ideas adequately?*
A. *Of course, yes. I live in America.*

FROM AN INTERVIEW WITH AN EXILE

The only problem is
they don't think much
about us
in America.
That's where Manila's
just as small as Guam is:
dots
on a map, points east,
China
looming up ahead. Vietnam
more popular
(because of that war).

They don't think much
about
expats, either:

Until they stink up
their apartments
with dried fish.
Or worry those
next in line at the fish shops
—that's where they insist
on getting
fish heads
Along with the fillet: "They're good
for soup, you know."
But distance helps—
all the same.

That's what it is—it's all the same:
so we hit the *New York Times*
and get
a curdled editorial.

Who cares?
The *Washington Post* can say as much
and the Potomac still
won't be changing course.
It's here, back home,
where the curdling
begins; where the minds can melt
like so much cheese.

10

Family Animals

"DID I EVER TELL YOU about the dog I had in the Philippines?" my father asked me when I was younger.

As a boy, my father lived in Tondo, the most densely populated area of Manila, infamous for its slums and high crime rates. Before it burned down, his family lived in a house above their *sari-sari* store, where they sold prepared foods, snacks, soda, and other convenience items. You could buy single cigarettes and sticks of gum, a dose of aspirin, or a packet of shampoo good for one wash. When he shared stories about his childhood, my American sensibilities were always shocked.

One day, a street dog followed him home and joined the other dogs already living in his family's yard. The dogs didn't have names; they were all called *aso*, dog. "Our dogs were not for petting," my father explained. "They were low-tech burglar alarms and garbage disposals."

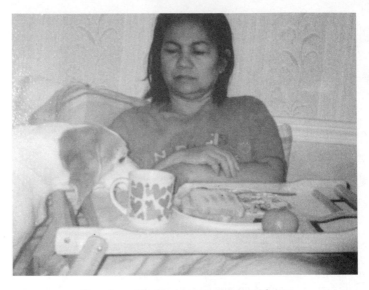

*Grace's mother Norma enjoying breakfast in
bed with the family dog, Sashi.*

But this dog was special. Totoy named his dog "Lucky," after Lucky Strikes. This detail still astounds me: at eight years old, my father had a favorite brand of cigarettes.

Totoy threw sticks and Lucky would fetch them. They would wrestle and Lucky would clamp down on his arm, but always gently, without breaking the skin.

Totoy's parents didn't hug him or say, "I'm proud of you, son." They didn't kiss his forehead when he was feverish or celebrate his birthday with cake and gifts. Those were for the rich. Life was tough and you didn't do your children any favors by softening them with encouragement and physical affection.

Lucky wagged his tail whenever Totoy approached. For the first time in his life, Totoy felt loved with abandon.

One night, a jeepney full of rowdy, drunk men slowed down in front of Totoy and his dog. A man reached a hook fashioned out of a pole and a bent clothes hanger out of the window of the jeep. He caught my father's dog by the neck and pulled it through his window.

"I don't get it," I asked. "Why did they want your dog?"

"What else for?" my father said. "To eat."

I shook my head. "Dad, they stole and ate your pet. You were just a boy. That was mean."

"It wasn't mean." He smiled. "It was meat. Dogs are meat the same as pigs, cows, and chickens, and the men were hungry. And drunk."

This is a trait I've picked up from my father. How to tell yourself a story in order to continue.

He liked telling this story, especially after receiving a vet bill for Sashi, our family dog. "Jesus Christ, why does the dog need to get her teeth cleaned?"

My father's teeth had been replaced with dentures in his twenties, precisely to prevent dental bills. He'd warn, "Be prepared. If this dog ever gets seriously ill, that's it. She's not having surgery or cancer treatments or diabetes shots. She's a dog, for God's sake."

I'd sometimes hear my parents fight about Sashi's expenses. She required specialty food, venison, for sensitive skin and didn't even sleep in her monogrammed beds from L.L. Bean. "Sashi is part of the family," my mother would say. My mother's devotion to Sashi was surprising considering her tendency toward germophobia. She is a woman who, when we were children, brought her own cleaning supplies to motel rooms so she could clean the bathroom before we used it. To this day, she carries hand sanitizers, cleaning wipes, and even toilet seat covers in her purse. She has the nose of a bloodhound and it's impossible to walk beside her down a city street on a summer afternoon without her finding an offensive odor to zero in on. When she gets onto a scent, she crinkles her nose and says, "Disgusting." She starts sniffing deeply and makes a face. When I ask her what's wrong, she points to where someone urinated on the street and makes a convincing argument about whether this someone was a cat, dog, or human. She takes these odors personally, as if whoever spilled the fluids of their bodies onto the sidewalk did it to make her ill. I tell her to ignore it. "Don't pay attention and you won't even smell it," I advise her. "I can't help myself," she says. I believe her.

She grew up with dogs, cats, and chickens roaming in her courtyard, but she did not consider them pets. As children, we were not allowed to touch our friends' dogs and cats and were scolded to move away if the pets tried to lick our legs or hands. My mother said they were "full of bacteria." But when Sashi joined our family, she ate from our fingers and licked our faces.

"She's a dog," my father would answer.

"This is America," my mother would counter, as if that made everything clear.

*

86

Rudyard Kipling's 1899 poem, "The White Man's Burden: The United States and the Philippine Islands," encouraged the U.S. to follow the lead of Britain and other European nations that had become imperial powers: "Take up the White Man's burden / And reap his old reward: / The blame of those ye better / The hate of those ye guard." This "White Man's Burden" became the euphemism for imperialism, which Filipinos embodied. It's a silly thing to think, but before I met my husband and had white boyfriends, I could not get the thought out of my head that I was a white man's burden. I dated two white men in the military and I wondered if people saw me the way I saw myself, a reflection of the documentaries I had seen about the U.S. military bases in the Philippines, the prostitution, and the Amerasian children forgotten and left behind. In college, I was constantly refracting myself through multiple mirrors, wondering who I was perceived to be by others, how I perceived myself. When I learned about "double consciousness" from W. E. B. Du Bois, I was relieved to read I was not the only one who felt this way.

Growing up, the consistent joke I heard comedians make about Filipinos was that we ate dogs. No insult felt worse than being called a dog-eater. Even though I'd never done so myself, I felt the shame of this practice tied to my body. Some animals were acceptable food sources, while others made you savage.

Perhaps this way of characterizing Filipinos began when we were displayed in living exhibits during the 1904 World's Fair in St. Louis. These human zoos were evidence in support of the U.S. colonization of the Philippines. The Philippine village was reconstructed over forty-seven acres at the fair and was a very popular site. I found the scrapbooks of visitors to the fair in the Missouri State Archives; among the many images and newspapers clippings about Filipinos, I found a photo of my great-grandfather, Captain Pedro Navarro.

One lasting legacy of the exposition, besides the invention of the ice cream cone, was the belief that your dogs were not safe with Filipinos around. My great-grandfather was one of those Filipinos at the fair, although he wasn't confined to the

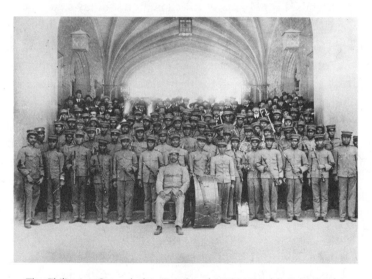

The Philippine Constabulary Band at the 1904 World's Fair. Grace's great-grandfather, Pedro Navarro, stands in the front row second from the left holding a piccolo. Seated front row center is African American Lieutenant Colonel Walter Howard Loving, founder and director of the Philippine Constabulary Band for forty years until he was reportedly beheaded by Japanese soldiers during World War II. Photo courtesy of the Missouri Historical Society, St. Louis.

areas where "the natives" performed their foreign cultural practices; instead, he marched in the Philippine Constabulary Band with his piccolo. He was the ideal outcome of U.S. colonization: Christianized, educated, military. The embodiment of colonial success. But all that mattered, at least in the American imagination, was what Filipinos did to dogs. When I visited St. Louis to learn more about the Filipinos at the World's Fair, a man at a museum gift shop whispered to me, "They ate dogs." Over one hundred years later, this is the story about us that persists.

*

There are stories my father doesn't like to revisit. Recently, as I was recounting a story about my childhood in the car, he slammed his elbow into his seat and shouted, "Fine! Everything is my fault. Just stop talking about the goddamn chickens."

When I was in the third grade, we had an incubator at school where we hatched chicks. At dinner one night, I told my father about the chicks, the marvel of the shell cracking and watching the slimy, gray creatures emerge. "I didn't know you were interested in chickens," he said.

A few weeks later, as an Easter gift, my father brought home five live yellow chicks, one for each of us. We were ecstatic. He never bought us gifts; to him, birthday cards and wrapping paper and stuffed animals were a waste of money. But real animals had a purpose. We named them. Mine, the only male, was Roostie.

In the covered area under the porch, my grandfather Tatang, who had recently come to live with us, built a cage for the chicks.

I overheard my father talking in Tagalog to my grandfather. My grandfather could sell the eggs and earn his own money for his cigarettes and beer. They had big plans: fresh eggs, mating, more chickens, more eggs. My grandfather held out his arms and measured where the other cages would go.

My sisters Tessie and Ann and I also had big hopes for our chicks. We would train them to do tricks, teach them to jump over sticks, and show them how to write their names by pecking in the dirt. On sketchpads, we designed elaborate costumes: cheery hats and silk-backed vests, four wedding veils and one black bow tie. They were our first pets—if you didn't count the short-lived tadpoles my older sister Tessie would collect from mud puddles or the cockroaches I'd play circus with when I was younger. After school, we raced off the bus. We chased our chicks in the backyard; we let them crawl onto our shoulders. We didn't mind when they peed on our hands—we just wiped away the mess on our pants.

But soon, the chicks got bigger, less yellow, and less cute. They still hadn't learned to jump on command and they scratched our arms. We attempted to tie toilet paper veils to the chicks' heads, but they wouldn't stay on. As their feathers turned red, we lost interest. And the hens never laid a single egg. Over the summer, we lost three of them. A dog or a coyote, maybe a raccoon. Around Halloween, another went missing. My father thought teenagers had gotten to it. Now only Roostie was left.

My mother was in the hospital for an elective surgery and was expected to be gone a week. It was something that today would be treated as a minor procedure, but back in the 1980s, my mother seemed to need minor surgery for something or other every year. We weren't privy to what she was getting done, and if asked by an adult, we were told to say that she was getting her knee fixed. I have a theory that she needed a break from us five children and her work at my father's clinic. Maybe she wasn't even in the hospital, but at a tropical resort somewhere by herself sipping frozen drinks. We kids took her for granted—the work she did that was undone daily—but once several days passed, we were desperate for her to return. My father only had one or two specialties that he served us, boiling hot dogs in tomato sauce and opening cans of sardines. We had to pack our own lunches. The bathrooms were filthy by the time she returned; our dirty clothes piled high. My father had sent my two youngest brothers, who were not in school yet, to stay with a neighbor.

"It's starting to get cold," my father said to me.

"Uh-huh," I said.

"Your rooster is all alone now."

"Yeah."

"Do you still want it?"

"Roostie? I guess not," I said. In truth, I didn't care for the rooster much anymore. He did seem lonely in his cage. Maybe my dad knew someone in the market for a pet rooster.

That Sunday, my father asked me to chop some onions and carrots. I tied my mother's apron around my neck and stood on a stool while I chopped the vegetables. I crushed cloves of garlic with the marble pestle and peeled away the paper. I hummed my mother's favorite song, The Carpenters' "Rainy Days and

Mondays". My father came up from the garage and retrieved a bowl, some rags, and a garbage bag. "You're a big help while your mother is away," he told me. He didn't exactly smile at me, but he did nod approvingly.

"Thanks," I said. Maybe I was finally supplanting Ann, my youngest sister, the favorite child, whom he had nicknamed Precious when she was born.

I went to the garage to ask my father how much rice to cook. On a workbench, my grandfather was squatting, smoking a cigarette and ashing on the cement floor. My father leaned against the wall, his fingers closed around the neck of a hatchet. Their eyes followed something whirling in the middle of the room, running in circles. Roostie's head lay on the floor. I watched his body slow down, stumble, and drop. His legs and wings twitched. I couldn't speak. I ran upstairs to my sisters.

*

Dinner was delayed that night and we were starving, but when the steaming bowls were finally put in front of us, we refused to eat.

"I'm not eating that," Tessie said.

"You are," my father said.

"We can't," I said. There was a leg in my bowl with pieces of cabbage and carrots floating in oily broth.

"You will," my father said.

We never cried in front of my parents, but that night we couldn't help ourselves. We sniffled and shuddered as we stared at the grains of rice strewn on our placemats. We stirred our spoons in the bowl but refused to lift them to our mouths. Our faces were red and miserable. My grandfather and father, headstones at the ends of the table, slurped their soup. My father shook salt into his bowl. (Since my grandfather's heart attack, we salted our food at the table.)

"When is Mom coming home?" Ann sobbed.

My mother was always the last one to sit at the dinner table. We would sit and wait for her to deliver the rice bowl and the chicken adobo, the fish head *sinigang*, or the stir-fry. After serving us drinks, she would pull up the stool from under the counter and squeeze herself into the corner between my father and Ann, onto the seat with easiest access to the kitchen.

"Yeah," Tessie sniffed. "It's about time she came home."

I tapped my spoon against the bowl's edge, saying nothing.

"We can't eat Roostie," Ann cried.

Suddenly, my father exploded. He banged his fist on the table and roared, "Eat, goddamn it!" My grandfather lifted his face and smirked at the open display of anger. Our misery seemed to please him.

As girls, we had the kind of relationship with my father where he only needed to raise his empty glass for one of us to jump from our chair and fill it. At mealtimes, we waited until he took the best pieces of meat for himself.

Since this was my fault, I dug my spoon into Roostie's boiled limb, which seemed slighter than the feather-covered legs that had run around the backyard. The meat was gray and stringy. My sisters followed my lead. As we lifted our spoons to our mouths, our tears pattered onto the soup.

*

Some years later, my father and Ann were visiting a pet store—or, as my father called them, "the free zoo"—while they waited for my mother to finish her shopping.

When they stopped in front of the fish tanks, my father looked at the price tags and whistled, "So much money for just an animal."

Then they moved on to the hamsters, which huddled together under wood shavings. At the sight of one of them running in the cage's wheel, my Ann squealed, "I want one! I want one!"

Although it was no secret that Ann was his favorite child, my father hesitated. He was a successful eye surgeon at this point, but still acted as if he were that poor boy in the slums of Manila, collecting fares by transporting passengers on his bike.

He calculated. Pet food, cages, wood shavings—but then he remembered the neighborhood girl who was adding to her college fund by breeding exotic rabbits in her garage.

"I'll take a male and female," he told the pet store clerk.

The clerk's voice cracked, "I don't think that's a good idea, sir."

"A male and female," my father repeated. "One cage."

He told the five of us that we should advertise to our friends and start taking orders for hamsters. "There's twenty in each litter," he said, "so each of you can sell four each."

The only information my father had on hamsters was the flyer that listed what to feed them and how often to change their water and wood shavings. Soon enough, the female, named 20/20 as an homage to my father's occupation, had fattened into a lumpy fur ball. We left 20/20 alone and only played with Trouble, the male. I woke up one morning to hear Ann's ecstatic voice, "She had the babies!"

As I began to count the pink jelly beans, Ann screamed, "The daddy is eating the babies!"

None survived.

"It's okay," my father told us. "She'll have another litter in about three weeks."

This time, we separated the male hamster right after mating. One morning, we awoke to find the new litter. Seeing the wriggling pink babies was like finding Christmas gifts from Santa or discovering an overnight snow had canceled school. We crowded around the cage, pushing and jostling each other to get a good look. The odor was strong and eye-watering. Suddenly, the female hamster ran from one end of the cage to the other, squashing the babies into the metal floor with her nails. None survived.

"I don't want hamsters anymore," Ann said.

Since female hamsters are in heat every four days and deliver a litter every three weeks, this cycle was repeated a few more times—but always with the same results.

My father returned to the pet store with the hamsters in separate containers. He wanted his money back. "If you pay us, we will take them back," the clerk said.

"They're not used tires," my father said. "This isn't an oil change."

"We have plenty of stock," the pet store clerk said. "We'd be doing you a favor taking them back."

Defeated, my father brought them home. We tried to avoid walking by the cage, but whenever we did our eyes would inevitably glance inside and witness the carnage. And the smell—of waste, birth, and death—was overpowering. A few days after the pet store fiasco, my father reported that it was very sad, but the hamsters had run away. "I think they're living in the backyard now. With the field mice and chipmunks," he said.

It made Ann and my brothers happy to imagine the hamsters running free in the tall grass and joining a community of rodents, perhaps attending tea parties and cookouts.

I never questioned my father's story; I was just relieved the hamsters were gone. When he finally told us the truth, we were out of college. For years, the lie had bothered him, a pebble in his shoe. During one of those rare times when all of us were seated around the same table, my father told us: He had dosed each hamster with a syringe of lidocaine, a local anesthetic he used as an eye surgeon, then looked away while they trembled, giving 20/20 and Trouble their privacy. He waited until they stopped shaking, wrapped them in sterile gauze, and hid them in the garbage.

*

The year I graduated high school, my father acquired our family dog, a purebred beagle, on a whim. Although he hated spending money, he could never pass up a good bargain, and a chance meeting with a breeder desperate to get rid of the litter's runt resulted in Sashi. The plan was that our dog, like my father's in the Philippines, would live in the yard, and in the New England winters, the garage. From the moment Sashi came home with us, she insinuated her way into our family. In the middle of her first night, Sashi woke my mother up, crying. My mother, half-asleep, picked up Sashi from her box and rocked her back to sleep in the same chair in which she had nursed my brothers. By Christmas, Sashi had a photo ornament on the tree and a stocking hanging on the mantle with her name written in glitter.

My father shook his head at the festive bandannas the groomer tied around Sashi's neck every few months. "You know, I've never paid for a haircut in my life," he said. "And now I'm paying for someone to clip a dog's nails."

Sashi was no saint: she would scatter the kitchen garbage and roll in horse manure after being groomed and pee on the carpet in front of our bedroom doors nearly every day. After stepping in a wet spot, my father would say, "Getting a dog was a big mistake."

On hot summer days, Sashi would escape from the yard to sit on the cool yellow line painted in the middle of the road. When Ann's then-college boyfriend Jorge first met Sashi, she snapped at his hand. "Don't take it personally," I told him. "She's bit all of us. Several times."

Even after he married my sister, Jorge would shake his head, "I'm not kidding. That dog needs to be put down."

My father pretended to hate Sashi, but things changed after his five children grew up and left home. Sashi began to sleep in the bed he shared with my mother, ride in the front seat with the window down on car rides to the town dump, and keep my father company as he took laps around the lake on his boat.

During Sashi's annual checkups, the vet always seemed surprised to find Sashi alive and well. She was overweight, and yet my father fed her table food as often as her specialty dog food for sensitive skin. After Sashi turned fourteen, the vet told us to expect things to go downhill, but it wasn't until Sashi turned seventeen that her health declined significantly.

We set a date to put Sashi down. I insisted on picking up a steak and cheese sub on the way to the vet's. "We're going to be late," my mother said.

I started to say, "They can't get started without us," but I kept my mouth shut. My mother carried Sashi on her lap in the front seat as my boyfriend drove.

Sashi lifted her head from my mother's shoulder as I unwrapped the white butcher paper, picked off the greasy strips, and placed the meat directly in the dog's mouth.

When we got to the clinic, my father was waiting in the parking lot. He reached for Sashi and held her stiffly. He leaned his head down to whisper in Sashi's ear. Then, he glared at my boyfriend, "Don't ever get a dog. It's a mistake."

After exiting the clinic, we found my father in his car, eating the other half of the steak and cheese. "That dog," he choked out. "It's so stupid. I didn't even cry when my mother died."

*

Later that week, as he was ripping out the urine-stained carpets, my father revealed what he had whispered in Sashi's ear. He was both surprised and ashamed. "How could I say those things to a goddamn dog?"

He said to the dog words he never said to his parents, words I've been waiting my whole life to hear: "I love you." And, "Thank you."

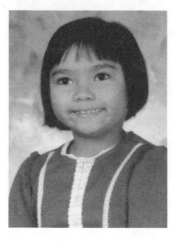
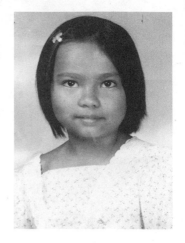

Grace in kindergarten, age 5.   *Grace in grade one, age 6.*

We are
happy to be
your new friends.
Happy Birthday

*A birthday greeting from Grace's first-grade class,
which she received on the first day that she attended
school in the suburb where she grew up.*

11

Monsters

ONE MORNING IN THE SPRING when I was eight years old, I woke up a puffy pink monster. My lips had disappeared into a mass of swollen flesh, my earlobes were triple their usual size, and my cheeks were throbbing hot.

I crossed my arms over my chest and scratched. I looked down and saw little red bumps that lifted themselves up and multiplied as I clawed at them, joining together to make flat islands, an archipelago of inflamed skin.

I'd always wished that I would go to bed one thing and wake up in the morning something else, but this is not what I had hoped for. The self I longed for was very specific: brown hair, hazel eyes, or blonde hair, blue eyes. It wanted to look normal like my friends. I wanted to look like the girls in the books I read and the movies I watched. I wondered if this was my punishment for praying for the wrong things. I was supposed to pray for world peace, for an end to hunger and suffering, but I was a selfish girl, praying only to look pretty.

*

My father's father, Tatang, lived with us off and on for several years. He slept on the sofa bed downstairs in what we called the family room, with its pool table and a television. Wanting to repay his father, who had only finished the third grade but found the resources to send him to medical school, my father would buy him tickets from the Philippines, feed him and house him for long periods, pay for his medical bills, and buy him Craftsman tools that lined the walls of the garage.

*

I didn't feel sick, just ugly. I was afraid to go into my parents' bedroom and show them. What if they didn't recognize me? What if I was too ugly to help?

My mother gave me Benadryl, but it didn't seem to make a difference, so the next day she brought me to the doctor. He asked us countless questions: had we changed our laundry detergent, our diet, our cleaning supplies, our soap, our shampoo, our conditioner, our lotion, our clothes? No, everything was the same.

None of the doctor's hypotheses explained the hives. But he was asking the wrong questions. It's not his fault. Who would have guessed? Several years later when I was twelve and my broken menstrual cycle hinted at a larger problem, another doctor asked about a symptom that seemed to point to a sexually transmitted disease, but the adults talked themselves out of it, my splayed legs between them. By then, I was a pro at dissociation. I could throw myself into the wallpaper or the nightlight at a moment's notice.

It didn't make any sense, the adults argued. I didn't have a boyfriend. I was too young. Again, the wrong questions.

Every spring after that, when my grandfather showed up at our home, I broke out in hives, my skin sounding the alarm of his return.

*

I remember the first lessons my mother taught me: The names of my body parts and how to pray. My *kilikili* was under my arms and my *kiki* was between my legs. Before sleeping, pray the Our Father so God will allow you to wake up again the next morning. Remember that your guardian angel is always with you. Thank your angel for keeping you safe. Pray the Our Father whenever you feel scared.

I was four years old when she told me, "Blood is thicker than water." When I asked her to explain, she said, "Family, blood relatives, are more important than anything." To this day, if my family needs me, I will drop everything to attend to them.

*

I remember who I was before my grandfather moved into our house. I was learning to add and subtract numbers with three digits. I raised my hand so often that my second-grade teacher would sigh and ask, "Grace, why don't we let someone else have a chance?"

By then I spoke English with a Boston accent. I played center forward on my soccer team and regularly scored hat tricks, three goals in a game. My dance teacher, a former New England Patriots cheerleader, taught me to stand on my head. In that position, legs straight up, balancing, I felt strong. I wanted to be the first lady astronaut. I wanted to travel the world in a hot air balloon. I remember hearing adults say, "What a happy girl" and "Look at that smile."

*

I was in second grade when my grandfather came to live with us the first time. When my father wasn't at work, he spent his free time with my grandfather. In the summers they worked on outdoor projects, and in the winters, they would wear their heavy coats and smoke in the garage, the door cracked open to let fresh air in and a space heater glowing bright orange between them.

My grandfather tilled a third of the backyard into an impressive garden and fed us with his vegetables. He grew green squash the size of baseball bats that hung from trellises. He indulged my request to burn worms and caterpillars and watch them shrivel away. He let me throw green potatoes from the garden into the fire so I could watch them explode. My father turned the garage into a workshop where my grandfather built things: two workbenches, cabinets to hold his new tools, a shed, and even a back porch and staircases. During the winters, he would carve wooden spoons. Even though my mother only needed one or two for cooking, the kitchen drawers, and then the coffee can on the counter she used to hold her spatulas and tongs, were crammed full of his hand-carved wooden spoons. They were silky smooth from his fine sanding and I liked to rub their heads against my cheek. My father gave up his den so that I could have my own bedroom downstairs, right next to my grandfather's. He offered to make me new furniture. I wanted pink everything, and he made me rosy bookshelves, a patterned side table, and a small, pink trundle bed of the sort I had read about in a children's book.

I can still recall the teacher who took me aside one spring day into the privacy of the coat room to ask, "Is anything wrong?" She said that I had changed.

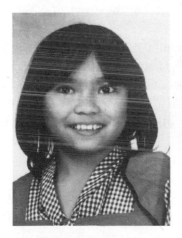
Grace in grade 2, age 7.

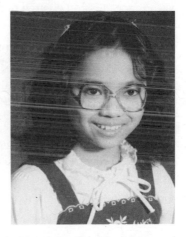
Grace in grade 4, age 9.

I remember all the pleasure had gone out of learning and school. I stopped showering and brushing my hair regularly. I didn't care if my clothes were dirty or my socks mismatched. Instead of following the math lessons and being the first to raise my hand, urgently needing the teacher to know that I knew the answer, my head was full of wooly clouds. I'd chew my nails and line up the white slivers in the groove of the pencil holder, pretending my nails were sails for boats that would take me away. I would fantasize about a hot air balloon that I hid in the attic. I imagined packing my suitcase with marshmallow fluff and peanut butter sandwiches and a doll, for company, who had her own little suitcase. The roof would crack open and I would climb into the wicker basket and rise into the sky away from that house.

My teacher asked if someone was hurting me, but I had no sense of my body's boundaries, and that to trespass them without permission created damage. Even now, I am discovering the extent of the injury.

If my grandfather had waited until a year later to start abusing me, once the mandated reporting statutes for suspected child maltreatment took effect, my life would have turned out differently. But at the time, I told her that nothing was wrong, nothing had changed. I didn't want my grandfather to go to jail. He would be so lonely there and I knew how crushing loneliness was.

To show you how malleable the mind is, how much it wants to believe a certain narrative in which family members don't hurt each other, during my evening prayers, I still prayed for my grandfather's well-being along with my other family members. As a child, the only way I could make sense of what was happening to me was that every night, I entered hell, and in the mornings, I was in heaven. There was a daytime grandfather and a nighttime grandfather, two different people in the same body. I told myself that the pain and sacrifice of my hell moments were required for my family's success. I never stopped to question if this was correct, if the kind of God we were worshipping as Catholics would ask this of his beloved people.

*

A few years after my grandfather's first visit, I was in the church parking lot with my father. He was picking me up after Sunday school. We sat in the front seat in silence. "What are you waiting for?" I asked.

He was staring at the young parish priest, watching the way he put his arms around the children climbing all over him, how he kissed them on the lips, lingering just a little too long. None of the other parishioners around seemed bothered by his affection. "Stay away from that priest," my father said. "Don't let him hug or kiss you. Promise me."

I did. My father didn't want me to be hurt that way, obviously, and he realized that there were people who could do that to my body. And yet.

Despite the whispers among the community about this priest, it wasn't until years later that I received a phone call from the church diocese. They asked me what I'd heard and seen about that parish priest. Some girls I knew had accused him of sexually abusing them.

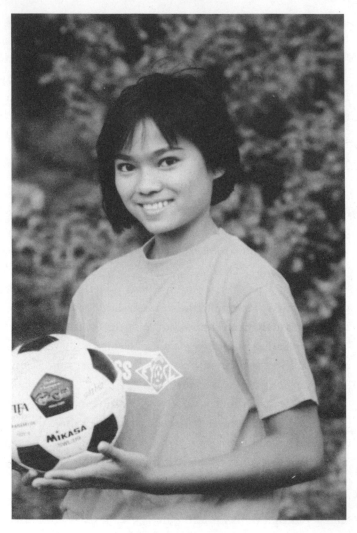

Grace in grade 8, age 13.

*

Eleven was my year of blood. I started my period, which ruined some of my favorite pants and skirts, most tragically the flamingo-pink skirt I wore once a week. I felt pretty wearing it, but after it became stained beyond repair, I had to throw it away. At the hem of this pink skirt, I'd been hiding a secret. What started as a warm spot on the skin above my right knee grew into a tiny pointed mountain over several days. It throbbed and swelled. I felt its heat against my palm. To touch it made me wince in a kind of ecstasy.

I was in near-constant pain, but I didn't tell my parents about this mystery on my leg. Or maybe I did tell them, but so quietly that they didn't hear me. My parents were so busy back then as new immigrants putting the pieces of their American Dream together: the small business, the house in the suburbs, the two cars. There were five us of children and no servants or supportive family like back home in the Philippines. I didn't want to be a bother.

When the pain got so bad that I needed to limp, I hid even that. I knew how to separate myself from my own discomfort, how to hide a wound, and I relied on this superpower often. The problem is that this maladaptive behavior separated me from other sensations, even the ones that I wanted to feel. I convinced myself that this was what being alive felt like.

At school one afternoon, I looked down at my skirt and noticed a wet circle spreading over the pink cloth. The mountain had become a volcano, erupting hot blood and fluid from deep inside me. I hid the tender spot with my notebook and then on the bus, I covered it with my hand.

When I saw my parents later that night, I lifted my skirt. "That's a boil!" my mother said. "That's very painful. How long have you been walking around like this?" My mother cleaned my wound and sprayed red medicine onto it. I sucked my teeth at the pain. "Aren't you lucky," she said, "to have a mother who is also a doctor?" She bandaged it with a large piece of gauze and followed up every day until the skin had healed.

"You should have told us earlier," my father said. But it had felt delicious to have this bodily secret. In all the world, only I had known.

*

The hives didn't leave a mark, and the boil became a puckered circle that I used to cover self-consciously whenever I wore skirts, swimsuits, or shorts. But that whole time I was nursing another secret wound—an injury that did not disappear or heal into a smooth brown coin. Instead, my life shaped itself around what was possible after its constant trauma.

My grandfather entered my life like lava, incinerating everything in its path.

12

Man in the Mountain

MY FATHER WAS EXCITED to show his parents America. There were dozens of photo slides documenting our visits to tourist sites in Chicago, Toronto, Orlando, Washington DC, Niagara Falls, New York City. We posed in front of signs and monuments with only my father, the photographer, absent from the photos. In one unusual slide, I sit alone underneath a wooden marker at the Old Man in the Mountain, a granite cliff in New Hampshire. Both Daniel Webster, a politician in the mid-1800s, and Nathaniel Hawthorne were inspired by the stone face and wrote about him. People flocked from all over to see him with their own eyes, and in 1945, his profile became New Hampshire's official state emblem. He is on the road signs, postage stamps, state quarters—the only U.S. quarter with a profile on both sides of the coin—and license plates, "Live Free or Die" written across his forehead.

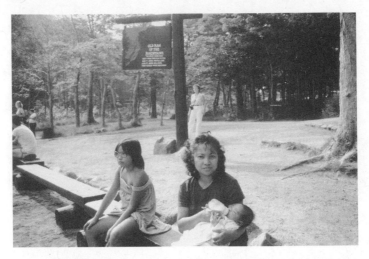

Grace sitting next to mother Norma while she feeds a
bottle to Jet under the Man in the Mountain sign.

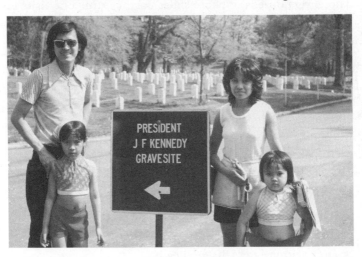

Grace with parents and sister Tessie at Arlington National Cemetery.

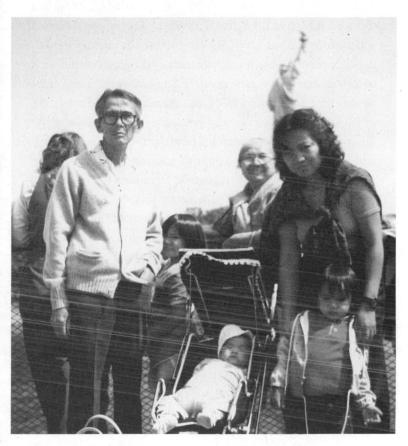

Clockwise from left: Tatang, Ann, Inang, Norma, Gerry, baby
Jet in front of the Statue of Liberty in New York City.

If you stood in the right spot, you could see him, the craggy profile of the Old Man's jagged face, made of five boulders cantilevered a thousand feet above Franconia Notch. In the picture, I stare into the distance clutching a paper bag. I earned what was in the bag from my chores, cleaning the floors. My father covered highly trafficked areas of the green carpet with industrial-strength plastic runners. Sometimes the metal tacks would come loose, and while I was cleaning, I would catch one in my foot. After every meal, I swept the linoleum floor in the dining room, capturing what fell from our mouths and napkins, and I used my allowance to buy cheap earrings and candy. The paper bag held a dozen candy sticks from the general store at the foot of the Old Man in the Mountain site. On the drive home, I lay down on the flatbed in the back of the green station wagon, unwrapping each stick—just enough to taste each unique flavor, butterscotch, cherry, lemon, root beer, and sour apple. I didn't want to share with anyone.

I was eight years old and my grandfather was seventy-one. I wore a straw-yellow sundress with inch-wide straps holding up the camisole top, with scalloped edges and a knee-length hem. I was still too young to wear a bra. Shaggy bangs hung over my glasses—my mother would trim my hair right before the start of school, my fourth-grade year.

That day, on our way home from the Man in the Mountain, my grandfather sat in the bench seat in the middle of the station wagon. My parents were in the front. Car seats weren't required; my baby brothers Gerry and Jet sat on laps. I don't remember where my sisters were; perhaps napping next to me in the flatbed. While we drove away from him, the Old Man in the Mountain watched as my grandfather casually draped his arm across the green leather of the bench seat. I ranked the flavors of my candy sticks in order: butterscotch, lemon, cherry, sour apple, and last root beer, which I did not like. He found the hem of my pretty yellow dress and walked his fingers over my knees and up my thighs. He breached the elastic around the leg hole of my underwear, which was embroidered with the day of the week.

Years later, I looked at photos of that day and was surprised to see my grandmother, Inang, posing with us. I don't remember her being there that day. All I see is him. I wonder now, where was my grandmother during all of this? Slumped asleep on the opposite side of the bench seat with her head against the window? Did she ever notice what her husband, always beside her, was doing to me with his arm draped behind her head? I don't have any confidence that she would have stopped him. For that to happen, she would have had to notice and see that something was amiss.

If you wish that something isn't happening, does that make it disappear?

Inang stayed back in the Philippines most of the time and was not with Tatang during his many visits to our house. She was useful and helpful to my parents when she lived with us, doing the laundry and cooking. But I can't say we ever had a conversation. There was a language barrier between us, but also something else. Usually she had her back to me, washing dishes or cooking or sewing. She would turn around and I'd feel like we were characters in two different movies, hers a 1940s World

War II-era black-and-white while mine was a John Hughes 1980s teen rom-com. As a teen snapping gum and wearing fluorescent-hued off-the-shoulder tops, I talked fast while my grandmother moved and spoke as if encased in invisible molasses. Her eyes were magnified behind her thick glasses and she often blinked at me silently, baffled, instead of speaking.

My father told me he felt special as a child because while his family didn't celebrate birthdays—that was for rich people—his mother scheduled the visitation of the Santo Nino to their house during his birthday. The Santo Nino, a dressed-up doll of Jesus as boy, stood on their altar in their home for one week, and they prayed the rosary in front of it in the hopes of receiving a blessing. Once he had established his practice, my father was proud to give her an eye exam at his clinic and handed her the prescription for new glasses. She looked down at the scribbled numbers and was so angry that she crumpled the square of paper into her mouth and angrily chewed it up. She thought her son, the one she had sacrificed so much for, had presented her with a bill for his medical services.

I later found out that my childhood white American friends who had met my grandmother called her E.T. behind her back, in reference to the 1980s Steven Spielberg hit about the alien who becomes a member of a troubled family. They said the brown color and flatness of her face and the shape of her head were just like E.T.'s. My grandmother didn't speak much English, and when she did, it was to utter two or three-word responses, like Spielberg's alien saying, "E.T. phone home." I suppose my grandmother's foreignness made my friends so uncomfortable that they had to make fun of her, but it is curious to me that they chose a literal alien creature to compare her to. The town I grew up in seemed so homogeneously white when I was a girl that I was surprised by the many passionate debates between what I considered simply white people, arguing about how many fifths and halves Irish, Italian, French, and English they were. During my childhood in that town, a man with Irish ancestry marrying a woman with Italian ancestry tracing back to their great-grandparents, both of them practicing Catholics, was considered a mixed marriage.

I know barely anything about my grandmother's life, and our relationship was mostly pragmatic. She helped my parents by watching us and doing housework. I've asked my father and other relatives, but I can't get a handle on who she was. All I know is that when she stayed at my parents' house and slept next to her husband, my grandfather, twice a night he left her side and she never did anything to stop it.

*

As a girl, I thought that one of the reasons this happened to me was that I really wanted a grandfather. I had read about grandfathers in books and watched kind old men dole out wisdom in movies and on TV. My life had been full of relatives in the Philippines, but we were alone in the U.S., and my parents were slow to make friends. Before he started abusing me, my grandfather groomed me, as gently as he raked the soil in his garden. He was a quiet and undemonstrative man, which made me seek him out even more.

When I see the stone heads of Easter Island, I think of him. It was Easter season when he came to stay at our house for the first time. I used my allowance to buy him an Easter gift, a metal tomato cage. I had noticed him growing seedlings and had felt great pleasure thinking of a gift that would make him happy.

I know few facts about my grandfather Tatang's life: He was one of three children, a small family for Filipinos. Both my grandparents completed school through the third grade, enough arithmetic to figure pesos and centavos for their income. In the Philippines, my grandfather worked as a handyman, and in a spare room of their home, my grandmother Inang operated a sari-sari store that sold "loosies," single cigarettes and aspirins by the dose. Depending on the day of the week, she also sold hot food, which patrons ate standing up: on Tuesdays, bowls of *arroz caldo*, chicken and rice soup thick as sludge; on Thursdays, plates of *pancit*, fried noodles with bits of meat, chopped carrots, and shredded cabbage.

Despite my grandparents' lack of formal education, they understood its value. Almost all of their children finished high school. Some even finished college and became professionals.

My grandfather lived many years of his life as a colonial subject. He was born a decade after hundreds of years of Spanish colonial rule of the Philippines into the time of the American colonial period. He was a husband and father during Japanese Times. What he experienced during World War II scared him so much that long after the atrocities ended, he stored a loaded gun under the bed he shared with my grandmother in case the Imperial Army ever returned to the Philippines. Uncles

whispered stories in my ear about Japanese Times: the behead-
ings in the square that the villagers were forced to witness, the
cousin who jumped out of a second-story window, broke his
left leg, and still managed to run away from the soldiers, and
the notes baked into salt bread that my uncle Emil, as a boy,
delivered to the resistance on horseback. It was better to be
killed, everyone agreed, than to be caught alive by the Japanese.

My father had a sister and brother he knew nothing about;
no one mentioned them after they died. During a records
search, I found evidence of his brother. He had the same
name as my grandfather and died at age one. I imagine my
grandfather losing his children, the grief and loss. It's tempt-
ing to draw an arrow between cause and effect, but there is no
making sense of what he did to me. We will never know; the
people who kept the secret of those children are themselves
gone. As an elderly woman, my aunt started to remember them,
these ghosts of memory. She says that her sister wore a red dress.
Or was it that her skin was so red that the girl seemed to wear
the scarlet fever like a nightgown? Before she died, the girl in
the red dress was old enough to run around, to flit and disappear around the corner of the bedroom, out of sight.

My father's older siblings were invested in his success.
They helped pay his school expenses in the Philippines, and
if he skipped school to play basketball with street children or
missed class so he could spend an afternoon on a rowboat in
the ocean, he was punished. My father wears his hair long to
cover a scar on the back of his head where his brother broke a
glass soda bottle and opened his scalp. "They were watching

out for me," my father explained. "There was no safety net and if I failed, it would have been big."

My father was so terrified of his parents that in elementary school, he hired a couple of street vendors to pretend they were his parents for a meeting with the school principal. But he made it through high school, college, and medical school. My grandmother showed up to his medical school graduation, my father tells me, "wearing her teeth. She only did that for very special occasions."

Do my grandfather's years as a colonial subject explain him? Perhaps his trauma, among other factors, created a desire to feel strong and he became addicted, getting his fix from dominating bodies less powerful than his. And yet, none of this justifies what he did.

I experienced sexual assault as a force that separated me from everyone else. I am still surprised when I am noticed—I came to believe that I was invisible, that I could disappear at will. But it was the other way around. My grandfather disappeared me. Perhaps he did not even experience my body as separate from his, and therefore believed he had the right to touch my thigh as if it were his own.

*

When I reunite with people from that time in my life, I get glimpses of how they saw me and what they remembered about me. They saw me as smart, confident, talented, and happy. And that was true; I was those things, too. They probably noticed that I was quiet, but I always had a tight group of loud friends around me. My senior class voted me "Most Likely to Become Famous."

They did not know I was depressed and sometimes suicidal. They did not know that I could not sleep at night and when I did, I was racked with night terrors and nightmares that did not fully disappear until I was in my thirties. I was so sleep-deprived that I could fall deeply asleep during the five minutes between each class period, and even in the middle of a friend telling me a story.

I had trouble learning. I remember guessing on most tests and quizzes. Maybe the model minority stereotype helped—teachers assumed I was smart and let me retake exams and redo assignments. I was in a deep fog and yet, somehow, I graduated and went to college. At times the fog lifted and I felt a renewed sense of purpose and excitement. But outside those bursts of hope, my inner experience swung, pendulous, between dissociation and depression.

*

In all the years he molested me, I remember him speaking only a handful of times, once to tell me, as he pinched my chest, "You're developing."

One spring day when I was seven years old and my grandfather was seventy years old, I was playing with my younger brother Gerry. I had just changed his diaper on my parents' bed. It seems strange to think of how much responsibility Tessie and I had in taking care of our three younger siblings, but we knew how to feed them and change their diapers early on. There are photos of Tessie and me at a friend's house down the street with our baby brothers Gerry and Jet. We took them along with us on play dates when our parents were out working.

I blew a raspberry on my brother's belly. It made him laugh and I loved the sound of a baby laughing. My grandfather was sitting in the room with us, in the rocking chair that my mother nursed in. He was watching us. He was always watching, and this feeling of being observed is still something that I can't stand. If I catch my husband watching me as I'm washing dishes or cooking, I send him out of the room. I'm now able stand in front of people and teach, but only after I found a way to keep their eyes off me and on the board, the screen, their papers, or their classmates instead.

One day while I was playing with my brother, we stuck our tongues out at each other. The tips of our tongues touched accidentally. I said, "Ew," and then we laughed.

I think that was the first night my grandfather came to my bed. He never spoke much to me, so I remember what little he vocalized over the years. Right before he stuck his tongue in my mouth that first night, waking me up from a deep sleep, he said, "I know you like this."

This was the story I told myself at seven years old: I touched tongues once with my baby brother and gave my seventy-year-old grandfather reason to believe I wanted what he did to me. Nothing else could explain it. I always felt that what he did to me was my own fault.

*

What I experienced is etched into my psyche: my grandfather's tongue in my mouth, the stubble on his chin, the pad of his index finger stained yellow with nicotine, his jagged thumbnails, the cold stickiness of his groin. There's him lying on top of me, skin to skin, my cheek turned to the side.

When he lived with us—usually for a season or two before going on to another relative's house—he would visit my room twice a night. First, when it was very dark out and then, when the sun was coming out.

He'd stand at the side of my bed, near my head. He'd take my hand and put it inside his damp, warm boxers. Usually he'd be wearing OR scrubs taken from the hospital my father worked at. He would put his hand over mine and make me squeeze him. I'd close my eyes and try to go back to sleep, my hand in his, and eventually he'd go away.

At dawn is when he liked to kiss me. His chin and upper lip were rough with stubble. I'd wake up to his tongue in my mouth. It felt like a writhing snake.

There were also surprise attacks outside of the usual routine. I'd be cooking breakfast or dinner for the family and he'd trap me in the corner next to the stove. Or I'd go downstairs to the garage to call him for dinner and he'd press me against the storage refrigerator where we kept the frozen herring caught the previous month and the surplus vegetables from his garden. In public, he was always trying to hold my hand and caress my fingers. We must have looked sweet, a loving grandfather with his doting, respectful granddaughter. If they'd looked closer, they'd have seen his long thumbnail that he filed to a point and liked to scrape lightly over my wrist.

For decades, I dreamed I was choking—a pillow over my head, a hand covering my mouth and nose, hands around my neck, an invisible darkness that prevented me from breathing. I'd wake up thrashing, gasping for air. Perhaps I held my breath when he had his tongue in my mouth, maybe for so long that I passed out.

I took to sleeping on my belly to make it hard for him to turn me over, but he always prevailed. He pulled my floral nightgown over my shoulders and did things to me, whatever it is he wanted. Mostly it was repulsive, but sometimes it could be comforting, the warm feeling of his hands smoothing over my skin. But even then, I didn't want it. I know he tried a few times to get inside me. I can't scrub some images from my mind, the feel of his weight and the odor of him on top of me. My body did not want to allow him entry. His insistence, his pushing to try, was painful. I felt the gouging of an already raw wound, the heaviness of him on top of me making it hard for me to breathe.

*

This is what happened and happened and happened.

I was seven and he was seventy.

I was eight and he was seventy-one.

I was nine and he was seventy-two.

I was ten and he was seventy-three.

I was eleven and he was seventy-four.

I was twelve and he was seventy-five.

I was thirteen and he was seventy-six.

There is no paper trail to document what happened to my body, and I don't remember all of what happened. The sexual assaults spanned seven years with such consistency and frequency that I was not present for all of it. I doubt I'd still be alive if I hadn't found a way to escape.

*

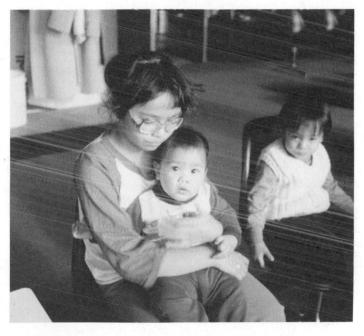

Grace with baby brother Jet on her lap and brother Gerry sitting next to her waiting at Logan Airport for a visitor to arrive.

It took a few years after the abuse stopped for me to be able to speak about what happened. Once I decided that I needed to tell, I worked up the courage for weeks, but every day was a failure. I knew I needed to tell—I was starting to come undone. Finally, at the last possible moment of a long weekend in January, I walked upstairs to my parents' bedroom. My grandfather was living at his daughter's that month and I didn't want him ever to come back to our house. After I told my mother, she hid her face in her hands and sobbed. She wanted to hug me, but the last thing I needed was someone else's sorrow. After I told my father, the first thing he said was, "Did he penetrate you?"

An arc of anger flashed through me so quickly that I almost didn't recognize it for what it was. I shook my head, but he needed to hear it.

"So he did not have intercourse with you?" my father asked.

"No," I said. Even then, I wanted to protect my parents.

I walked back to my room and got into bed. Telling had been so anticlimactic. All my father was curious about was the status of my virginity?

All those years, I thought I was protecting the old man with my silence. I expected my father to beat my grandfather bloody. I thought the old man would be killed. Every day, I thought I'd been saving his life.

My parents believed me. They did not seem very surprised to learn of my grandfather's behavior. And that's when I realized that he must have done this before.

*

As soon as I told my parents what happened, they warned me to keep it quiet. I can forgive this reaction now—they knew a story could destroy you. They had fled the Marcos dictatorship, where a petty grievance or accusation could get you assassinated. Even now, my father is still afraid of people finding out our secrets. While eating at a Chinese restaurant recently, my sister Ann's child Jada asked him about being a first-generation immigrant. Jada was studying immigration in school. My father whispered, "I'll tell you in the car," and looked around the room suspiciously, at all the other immigrants and descendants of immigrants eating dim sum from carts.

At the time, our immigration status was uncertain; Reagan's amnesty order had not yet been announced. My parents were preparing themselves in case we had to return to the Philippines along with our "anchor babies," my three younger siblings who were U.S. citizens. They claim now that they weren't worried, but this is part of our family's genetic code: to deny and dismiss.

After I told my parents what my grandfather did, my mother brought me to a mental health clinic. She told the intake person that my father was a doctor in the community and she needed assurance of confidentiality. It had already taken some work for my father to convince patients to trust him, a foreigner with a strong accent, for their eye care. We were one of two Asian families in my town at the time, and many of my dad's patients came from the church we attended, where he would hand out his business card every Sunday after mass during coffee and doughnuts.

Even as I write this, so many years after the fact, I worry about the repercussions of telling. I'm not afraid of falling apart by remembering, but I am scared of how this information can be used against me. Who will never speak to me again after I've told this story? Every time I write about this part of my life, I get a rash. I am covered in small itchy bumps on my trunk and arms and thighs. All the places he touched.

*

My grandfather was an unrelenting pedophile. He did monstrous things to three generations of his family. When I returned for the first time to the Philippines after being away for almost two decades, my excitement for the trip was shadowed by fear of my grandfather. He was still alive and I was still afraid of him. My mother assured me that he was bedridden many hours away from where we were staying. But she was wrong. Every elderly man on the street sparked terror in me. When his daughter, my aunt Ching, visited us, she asked how we could return to our home country and not pay our respects to her father. My mother took her into a back bedroom, closed the door, and told her the reason: it was because of what her father had done to me. After my aunt left, my mother told me that her response was "Too bad it was his own flesh and blood." I was floored by this answer. Did this mean his behavior was known? Had his predatory and abusive actions been tolerated when non-family members were violated?

*

Every relationship I've had has been impacted by my grandfather's abuse. My romantic choices were fueled by self-hatred. I had a boyfriend who said that I was so brown-skinned that he could only find me in the dark when I smiled. One told me I'd be a perfect woman if only I were waist high with no teeth and a flat head to rest his drink on. A high school boyfriend threw me away in a trash can near the football field for making him the punch line to a joke, and the metal sides were so tall I had to beg for his help to get out. Another boyfriend used a plastic knife to cut lines on my forearm moments before the lunch bell rang, and as I stared at the red letters on my skin during the next class period, I realized I was coming undone. My grandfather taught me I was not in control of my body and only existed for his pleasure. This lesson has made it difficult for me to connect with others, and that's the biggest tragedy, this feeling of separation. I have love in my life, but there's a part of me that hangs back from true closeness and connection.

Although she hasn't said it explicitly, I think my mother believes that what happened to me marks me for accidents and misfortune. There's just something about me, about my face, that makes people think they can do me harm. "You just look so nice, like an easy target," she tells me. "There are lunatics out there and you never know what they will do to you when you run into them." She encourages me to not to make eye contact with strangers or smile too much. "Don't appear so open," she says. "Look tougher."

I don't think she means to insult me. She is still atoning for what happened when I was a girl, which is why she pays special attention to me now over her four other children. She jokes that I am like her tenth and final grandchild and greets me with bags of new clothes and expensive moisturizers from fancy department stores. She showers me with the attention and affection she would have given my children, had I been able to have them. She invites me to accompany her on vacations all over the world. We've cruised on the Mediterranean, walked on a glacier in Alaska, and island hopped in Hawaii and the Caribbean. I've traveled with her to Mexico, Europe, and Asia. If she had her way, I'd never leave her house and risk hurt. I don't tell her that the irony of all of this is that the most hurt I've experienced was when I was living under her roof.

*

At various times, I've asked my parents and my siblings if they knew what was going on, and they've emphatically said, "No."

My mother asked, "Why do you think we would let him do that to you?"

I don't know. She's right. It doesn't make sense.

And yet, he did. He got away with it for years.

At one point, I found out that he had made a move first with Tessie. She was changing in her bedroom and the door was ajar. He stood in that crevice and watched her silently until she noticed him watching. She kicked her door shut and screamed, "Get out!"

He never tried anything on her again. I also learned that my grandfather liked to check his many grandkids' diapers for changing. If anyone was even concerned about this odd behavior, they told themselves what they wanted to hear: no, of course it's nothing.

One more detail: for at least a year, my sister Ann shared my bedroom and slept beside me in her own twin bed until I moved downstairs to my own bedroom, the room next to his. I like to think of myself as the hero who saved my sister from him.

*

Years later, the Old Man in the Mountain fell. In a video interview, the son of the first caretaker stands before the debris field where the stones fell, describing the collapse as "a terrible death." He said, "My heart was ripped out of my chest."

I didn't share his sadness. That face was tied to a memory of my grandfather. Even though he had died by the time the Old Man's face fell, I was glad to see him crumble.

I returned recently to see the Old Man in the Mountain site with my family. It was winter and we got lost, turning around and around on the snowy mountain roads. We stopped at the ski museum to ask for help. Finally, I hopped out of the van and stared for a long time at the bald spot in the mountain face where the Old Man's face once projected. I raised my arms to take a photo and my sister Tessie leaned her head out of the window. "Is this it?" she asked. "Why did we go to so much trouble to look for something that isn't here?"

*

This is how it ended. I had just turned thirteen and my grandfather was seventy-six. I was at my friend Kelly A's house and she was giving me a cosmetics lesson. First, the blue eye shadow and black eyeliner. Then the peach blush on the apples of my cheeks. Mascara came last. These colors were all wrong for my face—I was an autumn and she was a spring, according to a popular self-help beauty book women were passing around—but I felt hopeful that I might transform under Kelly's attention. Kelly was two years older than me and had been Tessie's friend, but ever since she'd been born again and started handing out kid-friendly pamphlets about the rapture, my sister had dropped her. I filled the vacancy. Besides, Tessie was busy most afternoons. She had to be ready to spring outside to fetch the mail or do some light weeding at the first sight of the paperboy's bike. Robbie was a tall high-school junior with cystic acne and he was kind to me even though I called him "Pizza Face."

We talked about our periods. She wanted to know if I had mine yet. I had, but it was unpredictable. At eleven, when I bled for the first time, I saw that first drop of blood on my panties, wiped it away and continued on to school. I had interpreted the term "period" quite literally to be a small drop of blood, the size of a dot. I was unaware that the bleeding would continue to pulse through me until I was sitting in a puddle of my own blood in a classroom of snickering fifth graders. The story of me walking across the classroom to ask the teacher if I could go to the nurse was the detail that everyone remembered about me until I graduated high school. I was that girl with the blood on her pants. When I got home, my mother gave me a cotton pad and then blocked the bathroom door to tell me cryptically that I now possessed a treasure that I needed to protect from those who would want to take it from me. I had no idea what she was talking about. I didn't need metaphors like the birds and the bees. I needed direct, scientifically accurate information about what was happening to my body.

"Everything is different after your period," Kelly said wisely.

"Why do people keep saying that I'm a woman now?" I asked. "I'm not taller. I don't feel older or different."

"Duh," Kelly said. "Because once you get your period, you can be a mother. And a mother is a woman."

I stayed still while she wanded black mascara over my lashes. She gently blew on my face to dry the paint and then applied another coat. And another. By the time I left for dinner and walked home, three houses away, I felt as if twin bales of hay rested on my face.

As I passed my next-door neighbor's house, I checked her picture window reflexively, looking for the Persian cat with the blue eyes. The cat was like a living, breathing cloud and it was the most beautiful living thing I'd ever been in the presence of.

Another Kelly, Kelly B, lived next door with the Persian cat. Kelly B had green eyes and thick blond hair that feathered naturally around her face. She was older than me by at least ten years but hadn't gone to college or ever worked. She had Problems. She once told me that if she ever got a cut or scrape, she would bleed to death since her blood didn't clot or scab. I imagined her spilling onto the ground through the slightest opening in her skin.

Being around this Kelly always gave me a queasy feeling. She showed up uninvited to my seventh birthday party as a mime and refused to speak until she'd washed off her face. White-faced and with a red smile drawn almost to her eyes, she wished me a silent happy birthday through robotic movements.

Once, I followed her into the woods behind our houses. She brushed aside some leaves and lifted up a plank of mossy wood to show me a plastic pail filled with tiny mildewed skeletons: squirrels, possums, rabbits, mice. Back then, I didn't wonder how those skeletons came to be in the bucket. I was too focused on their tiny jaws and eye sockets.

*

That day, Kelly's Persian cat was not in the window—it was on its back in the gravel on the side of the road. I almost stepped on it. Its limbs were curled as if it was in mid-leap, and a trickle of blood dripped down its chin. It was a statue of fear. I'd thought beauty was protection, but the cat's glassy sapphire eyes proved me wrong. From where I stood, I could see my grandfather in his garden.

Something happened inside me when I almost stepped on that cat. Somehow, for the first time in years, I felt clarity and certainty. I had just turned thirteen and I had a sudden realization that I needed to put a stop to what my grandfather was doing to my body.

A woman is a mother. This sentence clicked in my head like the sound of a pistol cocking.

I could not become pregnant with my grandfather's baby. No. I would not survive that.

That night, I felt excited to go to sleep for the first time since

I was seven years old. This was the last night I would go to sleep and be awoken by my grandfather's needs. I usually passed out with the lights on while reading a library book, but I clicked off my lamp decisively and closed my eyes to wait for sleep.

He could put his hands over my face and suffocate me so that I could not speak against him. He could call me a liar. I didn't care. I'd rather die early than live one more minute without authority over the borders of my own body.

The next morning, when his face came toward mine, I was ready. With both hands, I rose up and shoved his shoulders. Every cell of rage fired. He hit the bedroom wall and slumped to the floor. He quickly gathered himself to stand and closed the door behind him. He seemed both surprised and humiliated. That was all.

And my rage turned to joy.

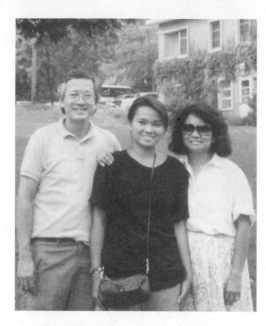

Grace with her parents before they dropped her off for her first year in college.

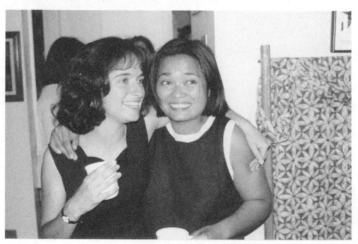

Joanne and Grace in their first apartment after graduation from college.

13

Unspeakable Sadness

I WAS A JUNIOR IN COLLEGE when I was diagnosed for the first time with major depression and anxiety.

I zombie-walked through that year and barely went to classes. I called in sick to almost every shift of my part-time job in telephone fundraising. Even the mindless, repetitive task of folding pledge letters and sticking address labels onto envelopes was overwhelming. My friends brought me meals from the dining hall in wet, collapsing boxes that the dining-hall staff decorated with smiley faces.

One night, my boyfriend returned to the dorm room to find me on the floor stabbing thick yellow phonebooks with his Boy Scout knife. He'd hidden the knife before he left for class, but I found its hiding place. I remember the urge to cut myself was so strong that I needed to plunge that blade into something substantive to keep myself from turning on my own body.

When I left the womb of the dorm room, I was incredibly anxious. There were too many people around and every interaction, even a brief exchange with a passing classmate, was unbearable. I was terrified to enter the empty hallways in the English Department building, sure that I was going to be attacked. When I used the public restrooms, the only ones available on campus, I willed myself to go as quickly as possible. I was certain someone had followed me in, was standing on the toilet next to me, and would reach over the top of the stall to bash me in the head. Years later, when my brother worked for the state medical examiner, one of his cases was a young woman who died in a public restroom in this exact way.

I have never been as ill as I was then, and every year since then has been an attempt to swim away from the dark depth of that illness.

*

Dr. B, the first psychiatrist I ever saw, was married to a Filipino. My parents had been friends with her husband Rick, also a psychiatrist, since our first years in Boston. When I was in high school and college, my parents seemed to spend every weekend playing mahjong—sometimes these games would go overnight, and I would wake up for breakfast and find the partygoers still sitting where I'd left them the night before, pushing mahjong tiles across the table. Now that my parents and their friends have aged and some have died, these mahjong parties happen rarely, maybe once every few years.

When I was growing up, I didn't interact with my parents' friends more than to greet them, but I was always curious about the white woman reading the book amidst all the noise of the mahjong tiles being shuffled across the table and eruptions of cheers and laughter at the end of a game. Like me, she didn't speak Tagalog, which meant being on the outside of the party—an experience I was familiar with—and she also loved to read. I never saw my parents read a book until their children were grown up and out of the house. Several years ago, I was looking through photos of my childhood in the plastic-sheeted albums in my parents' house. I came across a photo of my mother sitting with Dr. B at her wedding to Rick. I recognized another woman sitting next to them, Corazon Aquino, who a few years later, after her husband was assassinated, became the president of the Philippines.

By the time I disclosed to my parents what my grandfather had done to me, enough had changed in the culture around rape, sexual assault, and child sexual abuse—other survivors had bravely spoken up in talk shows and news specials, some high-profile cases had gripped the news for weeks, and TV dramas showcased the plight of affected people—that they knew what the next part of the story should be. Hearing people speak up about what happened to them changed my life. In 1983, I watched the two-episode arc of *Diff'rent Strokes'* "The Bicycle Man," and as earnest and cheesy as it is upon re-watching, that show started the wheels turning in my head so that I could eventually put an end to my own abuse. Later, daytime talk shows, especially Oprah's work, alleviated the stigma of being a survivor of sexual assault. Even though my father did not watch daytime TV, Oprah's story found its way to him and he treated me better because she told her story first.

*

"Do you want to see a counselor?" my mother asked me. After saying so much already, I could only nod.

My mother called Rick and asked to speak with Dr. B. The appointment was a few days later; my father canceled his afternoon patients and all three of us drove the hour's distance to Dr. B's office. I don't remember speaking after we entered. My mother answered Dr. B's questions and I nodded and my father sat silently with his chin tilted toward his chest, arms and legs crossed. At some point, Dr. B asked my parents to leave the two of us alone.

She wanted to hear my side of things. She said that as a long-time family friend, it was not appropriate for her to be my doctor, but that she would find someone closer to home for me to see weekly. I didn't know how talking with a stranger in an office could help me, but I trusted Dr. B. About my parents, she warned, "Don't have unrealistic expectations. Your parents don't have the vocabulary to talk about psychological issues. You will only be disappointed."

*

For most of my life, my faith in God was steady, but during this time, I did not feel connected to anything, including God. To be without God's light was another kind of hell. I preferred to be asleep, but when I opened my eyes to the darkness of my bedroom, the window shades always drawn, before I raised my head from my pillow, I started my childhood habit of praying, speaking to Jesus first and expressing gratitude for another day of life. But during this depressive episode and others like it that followed, I was deeply disappointed to find myself still alive. Even if I had wanted to talk to Jesus, my line to God had been cut. It is hard to describe nothingness and the pain of hopelessness and endless despair, but that is what I felt.

As a girl, I had grown up with a real fear of the fires of hell. I gave my weekly confession to the priest at the confession booth and every night prayed to be forgiven for my sins, even for the ones I had forgotten or did not realize were sins. I did not want to die with a sin on my soul and be vanquished to hell or languish in purgatory. Hell was a vivid place full of pools of boiling oil and fire everywhere you touched. I was taught to imagine a bad sunburn or when you accidentally touched your curling iron or a hot stove and to imagine that pain magnified a thousandfold: that was where you would go forever if you died with sins on your soul. I had a lot of time to think during that depressive episode. I came to the conclusion that hell was not hot, but cold. It was not an active, fiery landscape, but this: me under my musty and damp bedcovers, alone and without faith that there was anything good in this world to stay alive for.

*

During that semester, my mother told me that three of my aunts had been diagnosed with breast cancer and one with ovarian cancer. As a testament to how sick I was and how much pain I was in, I wished that I had cancer like them, so that my illness would be visible.

All I wanted to do was sleep. Unless I had to appear in class or at work, I was sleeping or trying to sleep. My dreams were intense even if I didn't remember the details upon waking, and once my eyes opened, the only thing I wanted to do was return to sleep. I did not want to be in what my life felt like. I did not want to be me. I'm amazed I was able to sleep so much. I hibernated like a bear, but without the hope of seeing spring. It's as if my body were catching up on all the sleep I missed when my nights were interrupted by my grandfather.

I was in bad shape, mentally and physically, probably the worst of my life. I thought about death every waking hour, about how much better my life would be if it was over, which, as I write this, I can see makes no sense. I had no motivation or desire to do anything—not to read nor talk to another human nor walk nor drink water. I just wanted to be asleep, to experience oblivion.

When I'm depressed, I despise the sun. I can't walk in the yellow light of day without feeling shame, irritation, and anxiety. I feel as though everyone can see and hear the darkness spinning inside of me. And at the same time, I'm full of guilt about my condition, about the narcissism and self-centeredness of depression. When I'm depressed, I become a liar. I pretend to be okay, but there comes a time when I can't sustain my lies. Depression makes me crave dark, warm spaces where I can hide from others and float in and out of a gray sleep—but this grayness thrives on isolation.

*

I needed help, but it took me a long time to call the college health center. I knew people went to the hospital for mental illness; looking back, I believe I would have qualified for in-patient treatment if I hadn't minimized my symptoms to the psychiatrist, a kind white man in a crew neck sweater at the campus health center. At the very least, I should have taken a medical leave from college and participated in a day-treatment program. But I held back during the psychiatric evaluation. I thought hospitalization for mental illness would smear my record and follow me from school to jobs to mortgage applications. Also, I didn't want to embarrass my parents. What would they tell their friends?

I also thought of my father, who believed that four sessions with his friend's wife was all I needed to be healed. During that first session with Dr. B, he told her, "We will do anything for Gracie. We'll come back here as much as she needs. Even four or five times."

As far as I know, my father, the doctor, has only seen a doctor twice in my lifetime: to pass the medical exam for immigration in the 1980s, and after he turned fifty when we children begged him to get a standard colonoscopy screening for colon cancer. Even though he's paid the expensive premiums for his own health insurance every month, he's always thought it a waste of time and money to go to the doctor if the illness is something he can address on his own with antibiotics or gargling warm water and salt. When my brother-in-law Jorge first married into the family, he joined my parents during one of their weekend mahjong sessions and sliced his hand accidentally. The party full of physicians quickly examined his cut, which clearly needed stitches, but they somehow convinced Jorge that waiting around in the ER would be a waste of time. Besides, mahjong is a four-player game, and if he left his seat, one table would have to stop playing. Jorge let them duct tape his wound closed and they continued playing mahjong. I believed my father when he said he would do anything to help me, but I understood why four or five sessions with a psychiatrist seemed extravagant to him. Dr. B was right in her assessment that my parents, at the time, did not know what therapy was and how it worked. My father didn't understand the damage that years of sexual abuse could do to a child's inner landscape. A home remedy of duct tape would not close that wound.

My father survived a childhood that we soft Americans would call abusive. My uncle John pointed this out at a family party ten years ago. My father's siblings were laughing and telling stories of their growing up, how they had been hit and punished, and Tito John shook his head and said, "That's not funny. That's child abuse."

As a small boy, my father had been tied up; hit with slippers, belts, and wooden paddles; had a glass bottle broken over his head. My father would smile and say, "Did I ever tell you about the time that I was so bad that my brother had to hit me over the head with a bottle?" Or, "You're lucky. We were hit with wood."

These allusions to childhood abuse were all remembered as funny stories from my father's boyhood in the Philippines, but

Tito John's voice suddenly reframed them. As horrifying and unfunny as these stories were, humor allowed my father to move his stories of suffering from the dark place where he hid them into the light. In turn, hearing his stories allowed me to connect the dots and see violence and trauma as on a continuum, and to understand that what had happened to me was not my fault. For most of my life I believed I was a bad person because something bad happened to me. I had to learn that I was not bad. I tell my story now in the hope that it will do the same for others, create an opening for their own stories and alleviate those feelings of aloneness.

*

During the years the abuse was happening, I knew implicitly how dangerous it was to tell on my grandfather. A story could get you killed, whether you were the person the story was about or the storyteller. My parents would often tell me to be careful of what I said, because "Even the walls have ears." You could not take a story back once it had been told.

Even though I didn't know the precarious immigration situation my family was in, I didn't trust the authorities, law enforcement, or the justice system. I was afraid that once the story was out of my control, anything could happen. A rumor could destroy an entire clan. You would be shunned, and no one would want to do business with you. I knew that my story was not mine alone, but that it would impact my blood relations, too. It was the only way I could feel powerful at the time: to know that I had the power to tell a story and to choose to withhold it.

For most of my girlhood, I told myself increasingly complicated and unlikely stories in order to cope: My grandfather would stop once his wife joined him from the Philippines. (He didn't.) If I let my grandfather abuse me, then he would spare my four siblings. (He didn't.) This misery would pay off and I would be rewarded somehow. (No.) If I lived through this, I would have experienced the one bad thing in my life and would be protected for the rest of my days from sadness, disappointment, and pain. (Nope.)

*

I didn't want my parents to have a daughter who was mentally ill, and neither did they. But the dual experience of the abuse itself, visceral and disgusting, and the denial of the abuse drove me deeper into mental illness.

I have engaged in various approaches to healing from trauma, including intensive individual and group therapy, sometimes multiple times a week. I have spent hours and hours of my life sitting across from other similarly hurting people in darkened, hushed rooms with tasteful, upholstered furniture talking about some of the worst of human behavior. With one of my first therapists, I was not even able to speak more than a few words each session, but she accepted where I was and allowed me to sit quietly and stare at her hairy succulent plant. I felt her caring, kind, and sympathetic presence. At the time, being seen by her was enough to make progress. I've read scholarly articles way above my head on the psychology of pedophilia, the lifetime economic costs of child sexual abuse, and studies such as the Adverse Childhood Experiences Study, and shelves of self-help books whose titles contain variations on the words "inner child," "courage," and "healing." I've attended self-defense classes for trauma survivors. I've made friends with other trauma survivors—we are numerous and common and would be friends without this particular history. Reaching out to other people and connecting, which is the exact opposite of how I felt when I was being abused, is why and how I am alive. All this work in healing has made it possible for me to have a life.

I recovered from that initial episode in college, but several times since then, I have sat across from a psychiatrist during a recurrence of depression and anxiety, unable to make eye contact, and answered a litany of questions about my mood, sleep, appetite, and energy level. I invariably leave these evaluations with various diagnoses of depression, anxiety, and PTSD, along with a grab bag of Klonopin, Paxil, Effexor, Celexa, Wellbutrin, Ativan, and Prozac to treat them. There are long periods when I take medication and then long periods when I don't need a psychiatrist's help.

*

My misguided wish for a physical manifestation of my illness came true. Years later, I had a double mastectomy, and upon the insistence of my mother, who wanted to take care of me, I convalesced at my parents' house—as it happens, in the same room where my grandfather made the comment about my developing breasts. I felt oddly relieved, I realized, that the part of my body my grandfather had most admired had been severed from me. The walls were painted blue now, and the wallpaper of my childhood—a girl throwing crumbs from her basket to geese—was gone. I used to stare at that wallpaper until I became the girl feeding the geese. I'd walk inside her hut with the thatched roof, put my feet up, sit in front of the fire, and wait for it to be over.

*

Several years ago, I accompanied Ann to the pet store to pick up food for her dog. In the parking lot, my sister hoisted the fifty-pound bag from her cart and handed it to me. I wrapped my arms around the bag of food, pressing my cheek against the laminated paper and hugging its weight—a serious, respectable, comforting weight. The bag started to slip from my hands and I dropped it gently into the back of the minivan.

"This is how much weight you've lost. It's like the weight of a second grader." My sister asked if I felt free now that I didn't have to carry that extra person around, that second grader.

"Totally," I said, but suddenly, I felt lonely and bereft.

For a little while after losing the weight, I'd felt like a better person, but soon, as my appearance and confidence improved, the attention from men began. The gaze from strangers made me want to fly out of my skin. Soon after losing the fifty pounds, I began a new project: gain it all back. I ate holiday boxes of Thanksgiving, Christmas, and Valentine's Day chocolates. I ate carbs after 8 p.m. I ate and ate until I had made the barrier I needed to stand between me and the world. Or perhaps, rather than the extra weight protecting me, I ate so that I could carry the second grader around to protect her, to give her an adult to hold on to.

I created my body in response to his. My destruction of this body isn't radical, but an everyday neglect. I don't sleep well or move enough. I eat too much of the wrong things and even too much of the right things. Sometimes I have trouble breathing, punishment for smoking in my twenties.

I once drew a picture of myself in which my head floats over my body like a balloon. That's where I really live, my head; my body is just the vehicle.

*

When I was a teenager, fit and tight, I recoiled at the nude bodies of older women, loose and lumpy, straining against their garments. When I was in high school, a woman in her sixties happened to change into her dress in a room I was in. I had not seen the real bodies of women before. She must have seen my face. She said, "Just wait until you have children and get to my age. You'll see."

I averted my eyes and said something agreeable, but I thought, *No. Not me. I will never let myself go like that.* And yet over time I've gained weight slowly and steadily. I've increased my girth and become solid and heavy.

I know I should be embarrassed of this body. I drape oversized clothing and dark colors over it, but I don't fool anyone. I know better than to wear horizontal stripes or sleeveless tops, but even when I was almost half my current size, I still tried to hide my body. During my college depression, more than once, family members walked right past me when they didn't recognize the person layered in tights, socks, a prairie skirt, a flannel shirt, sweatshirt, a light jacket, a heaver jacket, and a hat. They nicknamed me Bag Lady.

I still need a layer of padding between me and the world. The extra weight I carry is a cozy quilt, and anytime I need comfort, I cross my arms over myself. I am my own transitional object. I know there are consequences. I am too young to have feet and knees that ache this much. This is what a body can look like after it has been invaded.

*

During that particularly awful summer, my father offered his own story. As a small boy, he had been sexually coerced by a neighbor in exchange for candy. And he turned out fine, right?

"What happened?" I asked.

"That's it," my father said. "I told you the whole story."

"But what did the neighbor do exactly?" I asked.

"He gave me the candy," my father said.

Or while sitting in the car together, he'd offer, "Imagine that part of your life is a room. Close the door on that room and move forward."

I did try that. I said my father's lines to myself as a daily mantra, but what was hidden inside that secret room oozed through the cracks and doorjamb. It was so much work keeping that figurative door shut that I had recurring nightmares of trying to close and latch every unlocked door and window in my parents' house before the scary thing arrived. Sometimes the scary thing was a storm or a swarm of bees or a man, but I could never close every opening in time. My only escape from the scary thing in my nightmares was to jump and flap my arms and hope that I could suddenly fly. I was always amazed when I discovered that I could. It was such a relief to soar over my house and yard into the blue sky. After decades of nightmares, I practiced lucid dreaming. I read that you had to face the scary thing in your dreams. In one dream I turned around to face it, sure I would die of terror, and I shouted at the gray shadow and it melted away into smoke, into nothing.

About ten years ago, in the midst of a particularly bleak depression, my father asked me to follow him downstairs to his den. He pulled out a folder from the gray cabinet and handed me a typed letter. It was in Tagalog. "It's a copy of a letter I sent to my father many years ago," he explained. He read it aloud, in Tagalog, which I could not comprehend.

I wondered, with his third-grade education and near illiteracy, if my grandfather read this letter. If not, had one of my relatives read it aloud to him? Or did they spare his feelings and pretend not to know who he really was?

My father pointed to a line, repeating it Tagalog. "This is where I tell him: *I know what you did to Gracie. You are dead to me now.*"

With that piece of paper, he killed his own father.

After I told him what happened, my father cut all ties with my grandfather and wouldn't send money for his eldercare or his funeral. His family was angry with him. As an American doctor, my father was considered rich. His older brothers and sisters had invested in his success and he should have carried the burden of Tatang's care. Was my grandfather shocked that my father wouldn't have anything to do with him? What did he expect would happen when everyone found out what he was doing to me? Maybe Tatang never expected to be caught. Or maybe he had counted on raising children who raised children who always did what they were told.

Since sending the letter, my father's relationship with his siblings has never recovered. Something was severed that couldn't be reattached. You have to understand how radical my father's actions were: Filipino families stay tight. Vast kinship networks were crucial to survival during brutal times of poverty, wars, and colonization. Sometimes you must sacrifice yourself for the good of the family. I was afraid that my telling would change things and it did. I have heard whispered stories of who else was abused, but no one has joined me in solidarity. I know I'm not the only one he did this to, but I feel the lonely weight of being the only one so far to speak up. We stopped making the effort to see the larger clan and grew apart from my father's side of the family. I have always felt this was my fault. But now that their patriarch is long dead, what are we preserving with our silence? Who is left to protect?

September 5, 1990

Dear Bubut,

Remember that name? How are you? You may not realize it.
I miss you already. It is just a little comforting to
know that you are just two hours away.

It is the first day of school for the rest of the kids.

We are very proud of you. Do good in school and we will be
prouder.

Be careful walking around (I know you are careful but I
have to remind you anyway).

That orientation was well planned. We got home without any
problem. Mom was crying after you called Monday. She got mad
at me when I told her that there is no reason to cry. "You
don't understand how a mother feels."

Have you gone to the other colleges yet. When you are free,
take a dry run of the bus system there. You have an audition
on Sunday, right?

This is all for now and you take care. Good luck for this school
year. I love you.

Love,

Dad and Mom

*Grace's father's first letter to her, which he sent
when Grace left home for college.*

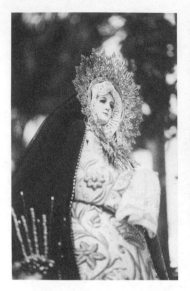

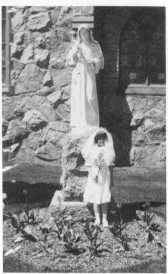

A statue of the Blessed Virgin Mary is paraded during Holy Week in Manila. Photo: Alonso Nichols.

Grace posing with the church statue of the Blessed Virgin Mary after her First Holy Communion at age 7.

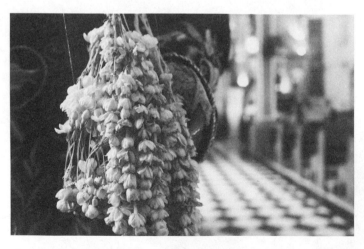

A string of sampaguita hangs at Barasoain Church in Malolos where the Philippines Constitution was drafted in 1898. Photo: Alonso Nichols.

14

The Bullet in the BVM's Crown

MY BELIEF THAT THE CATHOLIC CHURCH was a body I belonged to got me through so much of the darkness. That Jesus was the head of this body, that the Holy Spirit lived in my heart, that my guardian angel was always with me, and that the Virgin Mary and her husband Joseph were another set of parents. I was in constant dialogue with this voice that could be God, Jesus, the saints, or even the spirits of those who had died. A woman had taught me to pray as a habit. To open my eyes in the morning and have my first thought be Jesus; to close my eyes with my last thought, Jesus. On my birthday, even if it wasn't a Sunday, I should eat his body and thank him that he kept me alive another year. Without my faith, I don't think I could have kept going.

Every Sunday of my life I heard how Jesus had told his disciples to *eat this bread and drink this cup*. I kneeled on the pews, bowing my head during transubstantiation when the Communion bread became body, and stuck out my tongue to receive Him. At twenty-two, I had just graduated from college and knew that the Catholic version of God wasn't the only story. You could say I was experiencing a crisis of faith. On a pilgrimage with my mother to Lisbon, I frowned as I studied the glass case holding the Bleeding Host, a grayish circle of bread with a glob of red oozing from it. The guide told us that the blood type was the same as Jesus' and everyone gasped.

I wanted to believe. But I couldn't help wondering, *how did this wafer of wheat from the twelfth century had survived until now?*

The pilgrims remarked that I was such a good daughter to travel with my mother, but I feared those holy people could see through to the real me. I envied and coveted. I got drunk and high and enjoyed premarital sex. I sinned constantly.

Next, we traveled to Fátima, where in 1917, the Blessed Virgin Mary (BVM) had appeared as an apparition to three shepherd children. Thousands of pilgrims visited this site every year. I stayed behind when the tour group visited one of the children, now a cloistered nun. I explored the kiosks selling religious souvenirs. I dug through a bin of body parts molded in wax: legs, intestines, hands, hearts, and fetuses. I bought three breasts for my aunts with cancer and threw them into the pyre. It couldn't hurt. The wax breasts melted into a yellowish smoke that I imagined seeping into God's ears with my prayer, *Heal them.*

I stood at the edge of a marble walkway. At its end stood a Virgin Mary statue. In her crown was a bullet taken from Pope John Paul II's body, given in thanksgiving for surviving his assassination attempt. Pilgrims walked toward the Virgin on their knees. Some wore cotton pads; some tied bandannas or T-shirts around their knees. It was a long way, almost a quarter of a mile.

I didn't think, but knelt onto the path, scalding in the summer heat. I was surprised by how quickly the pain came. I distracted myself from those two burning points and moved forward. "Oh God," I sighed through my clenched teeth.

I wasn't asking for anything specific from God, but I was filled with a longing that everything in my life would work out. I thought of my mother at a convent hours away, writing my name on a slip of paper and handing it to a silent nun, perhaps the same woman who had set this place in motion.

Once the Virgin was close, I stopped. My body did not want to hurt in this way anymore. I understood what it meant to be flayed.

Later, I hid my wounds from my mother, but they stained my skirt. Even now, I'm ashamed. I had used my body to pray and made a spectacle of myself.

When I could not go on, a man and a woman appeared beside me. We didn't speak the same language, but they peeled me from the ground and lifted me. They held me under the arms until we reached the end. I felt I should kiss something: their hands, the Virgin's feet, the bullet in her crown. I was delirious with thirst and pain; what I remember kissing was hard and cool against my lips.

*

It was the reporting on the priest sexual abuse scandal in the *Boston Globe* that tipped me from practicing to lapsed Catholic. On January 6, 2002, the *Boston Globe* Spotlight team began publishing a series of articles, eventually over six hundred stories, about the Church's policies and practices that protected clergy who abused thousands of children. I was a believer for most of my life. I prayed the rosary. I attended mass, as they say, religiously. There were times in my life I would go every day: my Tita Alex told me to take Communion daily like a spiritual vitamin, and I did. I attended mass around the world. I could follow the rituals of mass no matter where I was or what language it was conducted in. This was a comfort.

When the Spotlight articles broke, I had been attending a church on the hillside behind where I lived. It had a statue of the Virgin Mary in the front. She made the news when she had started crying. Two gray streaks appeared under her eyes that no one could explain. But after the Spotlight articles, I couldn't attend mass anymore. And then the neighborhood church closed, like many churches did in the wake of the scandal. For a long time, I lost God, which was a terrible separation. Praying, meditation, and talking to God in my head is what had helped me heal through some of the worst periods of despair. I needed to believe that what I endured with my grandfather had meaning and that this sacrifice had a purpose. I don't believe those things anymore.

One Sunday when I was a girl, my mother brought us to hear Cardinal Bernard Law give a mass for the Filipino community in Boston. After mass, people crowded outside the church around the cardinal and my mother pushed me forward to kiss his ring. "He might be Pope someday," my mother said.

I did not want to, but it was too late, and the Cardinal knew what I had come for. He allowed me to take his hand and bring his ring to my lips as I bent forward. The gesture was natural to me, a bowing very similar to mano po, once to the Spanish colonizers and now to our elders, which generations of people who came before me practiced. This was the time during which Cardinal Law had been shielding priests who were sexually abusing children. For decades, Law protected these men, rather than the children who had tried to speak up about their injuries. How many lives would have been altered, how much trauma avoided, had he raised an alarm decades earlier?

I return to church sporadically for funeral masses, holidays such as Easter and Christmas with my parents, and to celebrate the First Communion of some of my nieces and nephews. Every time the young boys and girls, dressed like child grooms and brides, march up the center aisle with their hands pressed together, I am moved to tears. They glimmer. I remember receiving my first Communion. "Don't bite Jesus," my CCD teacher warned. I let him dissolve on my tongue. I watch the children open their mouths before the fingers of the priest, baby birds hungry for their spiritual food, and I wonder how many of these children we will fail.

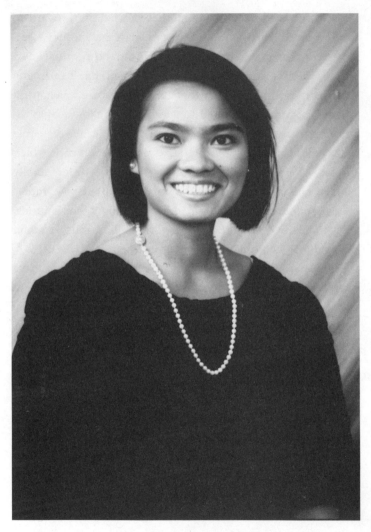

Grace's high school senior portrait.

15

Yellow Children

MY COLLEGE ACCEPTANCE LETTERS came with invitations to visit campus before making my admission decision. My friends did not get these invitations. These programs were for students of color. I was invited by offices for minority or AHANA students, an acronym for individuals of African, Hispanic, Asian, and Native American descent, to spend a day on campus attending classes, meeting with current students, and eating in the dining halls.

At one college, a Harvard professor, Sara Lawrence-Lightfoot, gave a speech. I don't remember a single thing she said, I only remember what I felt, which was awe. I had only encountered professors, in real life and the movies, who were white and male. Professor Lawrence-Lightfoot was a revelation. I wanted to be her. I thought college would be like this: full of women of color standing in the front of lecture halls addressing mostly students of color. I didn't know how rare this experience was.

In my predominantly white suburb, I never met a teacher or administrator of color, not even a substitute or janitor, during my twelve years of elementary and secondary school, until one day, halfway through high school, an Asian American guidance counselor showed up. The big joke, until he married one of the science teachers, was that I was going to marry him. I'd endured—and hated—these kinds of jokes since we moved to the U.S. There was one other Asian family that lived in my town, also from the Philippines, and they had a son in my grade. The jokes had not evolved much since then.

Sometimes I could forget who I was, that I wasn't white. I acted as if I was the same as my girlfriends. I wore the same bright blue eye shadow and sprayed Sun In over my black hair as I tanned at the beach, which bleached my hair the color of a mushy pumpkin instead of the sun-kissed blonde my friends idealized. I was like everyone else until I walked by a plate-glass window or bathroom mirror or saw a photo of myself with my friends, who in that image became my white friends.

During the admissions process, my classmates and even some parents and teachers told me I was lucky to be a minority student. I would have an advantage. Too bad I wasn't Black or Hispanic, though—then I'd have had an even surer shot at one of the placements promised to minorities in elite colleges. The subtext, which no one said aloud, was that we did not deserve these spots that we were taking from white students who worked so hard and earned it more. I got the message.

Not only was I insulted by how breezy and casual people were with their racial comments, but I was deeply hurt. I had lived in this community since I was five years old, but I was still other, foreign, and suspect. And yet, growing up, when I heard people make disparaging comments about Mexicans, Black, Jewish, and even Chinese people, I didn't speak up. I distinguished myself from those people by saying, at least in my head, that I was from the Philippines, not China, as if that made any difference. What mattered was that I was not white, whatever that meant. This happens all over our country. Every year, the students of color I teach at one of these elite colleges tell me that they heard these same comments from people they thought were friends.

These ideas have a long life. My students carry them into my classroom. They tell me they don't deserve to be on campus; they feel profound guilt. They believe the rhetoric—that they took the place of someone who deserved it more. The implication is that this someone is white with better grades and more talent. This guilt and self-doubt impact their performance, but also spoil their happiness in what should otherwise be an exciting part of their lives.

As a college hopeful, I returned to my suburb from those recruitment programs altered every time. The phrase "micro-aggression" was not yet prevalent, but at the time my eyes were opened to all the ways in which I'd been experiencing them. And I was starting to turn this anger outward instead of blaming myself.

After the college visits, I started to refer to minorities as people of color, adopting the term from the students I had just met. The first time I dared to say this aloud to a white person, I was talking to a school administrator explaining why I decided not to attend his alma mater. "I want to go to college with more people of color," I said.

It was a warm late-spring day and he was wearing a white short-sleeved Oxford shirt. He tipped his head and his glasses slid down his nose. He blinked at me. He pressed his finger against the skin on his forearm. "Look," he said. "My skin is darker than yours." I placed my bare arm next to his. Yes, his skin was tanner than mine, perhaps from weekends playing golf. "I'm no more a person of color than you are," he said.

I felt overwhelmed and embarrassed. I agreed with him. I'm still mortified at how I acquiesced. At the time, the development of my racial identity was still in the fetal stage. Maybe I wanted him to be right. I also wanted to believe that my life would not be impacted negatively by race. Even now, I wish this were true. As a high school senior, I had no clue how to talk about race to white people. I still have no idea how to navigate that minefield.

A week after this encounter with the administrator, a friend told me that some mothers of my classmates were talking about me. They thought it was improper that I was dating a white boy. One mother was worried about my future unborn children. "What will they be? What is a half-yellow and half-white anyway?" she asked.

I didn't want to be hurt, but I was. I walked down the school hall with tears streaming down my face. These women had watched me grow up in our small town, a place I felt I belonged to, and yet, perhaps all along, I had been only a foreign exchange student. I wish I could have responded then: Lady, if I had children, they'd be human. Just like yours.

As the weeks rushed toward high school graduation, I just wanted out. I was done. There was another world out there, one where I wouldn't have to pretend I was someone else. During a classmate's graduation party, my best friend Becca made a comment about Orientals, and I surprised myself by asking her to stop saying that word. "We're not rugs," I said. "Call us Asian American."

Even though I was the only Asian person at the party, I said "us"—I felt connected to a larger community of Asian Americans and other people of color. I was certain it existed. This was a "we" that my friend could not participate in—for once, it felt good to be inside a group. The room quieted around us. My friend's face pinkened as if I had slapped her cheek. Never in the dozen years we'd been friends had I complained in this way. I wondered if this would be the end of our friendship. We were actually standing on an Oriental rug.

We'd been best friends for most of our lives, a connection that sparked on the playground over a book, S. E. Hinton's *The Outsiders*, and that burned brightly through the highs and lows of growing up. We openly referred to each other as soul mates, kindred spirits, and "bosom friends" like Anne Shirley and Diane of Lucy Maud Montgomery's *Anne of Green Gables*. I had never met another girl like her, full of fire. As a little girl, Becca told her father off more than once, and he did not strike her or shout her down. He let my friend exist in her anger; it was liberating to watch. We had lots in common: books, music, movies, and talking about our dreams, our families, boys. I escaped often to her house, a big Victorian full of books and freedom. During mealtimes at my house, I was told to be quiet and eat, but her parents made conversation over dinner and asked our opinions. Once Becca told me, "I don't see race. I think of you as white," and I pocketed this gem, bringing it out to polish whenever I felt my difference as an Asian face in a mostly white suburb.

A person did not even need to use that word, Oriental, for me to feel that very particular kind of humiliation, shame, and diminishment that comes with racism. As Catholic Filipinos, we attended Sunday Mass faithfully every week, which sometimes meant sitting behind a white family whose small children would turn around in the pew to stare at us, then pull back the corners of their eyes. My family ignored them. We pretended even to each other that we didn't see them asserting their power. These children could barely speak, they were so young, but they already knew how to communicate their whiteness. They knew what fun it was.

I never heard Becca use that word again, which I appreciated, and we stayed friends through college, even though we didn't attend the same school, and after, as we began our adult lives. Our friendship had already endured for a quarter century and I was sure we'd be friends forever. She fantasized about us buying houses next door to each other and getting pregnant at the same time so that we could share new experiences simultaneously and then raise our children, who would also be best friends, through the stages of life.

Race wasn't relevant in our friendship. And yet. After graduate school, I visited my friend at the brewpub where she waited tables. It always stank of yeast and fried batter. She was at a difficult point in her life. We were a few years out of graduate school, long enough after college for the foreboding sense that our childhood dreams might not come true to sink in, but too soon to realize that our dreams might change. As a waitress, she felt invisible for the first time. "It's like they don't even see me as a person," she complained. "I'm just the help."

Finally, she understood. I'd always felt like a liar trying to convey this feeling. When I waited in lines, sometimes cashiers looked behind me to find the next customer. Police officers and others in authority would ask me if I could speak English if I paused before responding. My friend, in her pain, repeated something I had heard her say before, some version of: *You get all the breaks as a minority. And there's nothing left for regular people like me.* I sat across from her and dipped my pretzel in beer cheese. It was true. I was doing what I loved. I was living on my own and paying all my bills. Becca, off and on, was still living in her childhood bedroom.

She unfurled silverware from a black napkin onto the table. She had spent the morning making roll-ups before the restaurant opened for lunch. And then she repeated something that she and her coworkers noticed. The gist was that Black people didn't tip well, and the servers resented this. "Well, it's true," she said. "All the other servers say the same thing." She waved her hand in their direction—they were white. Those who bussed the dishes and cleaned the restrooms were not.

She said it so casually, oblivious of inflicting injury. Did she see me as an honorary white person? Had she forgotten that the man I was going to marry was African American? Or did she feel a thrill to remember this fact and say it anyway?

When I see how his skin is read, I feel a line drawn inside me. People cross the street to avoid him. Sometimes we take care of my sister's little feisty dog, and when Alonso returns from walking him, he reports how strangers smiled at him and sometimes stopped to pet the dog. "When I have a dog with me, it's like I'm living in a different world," he says. The kind where he is not constantly read as a threat. When he takes a flight, he dresses as if he's attending a wedding. Often, he can't hail a cab. During his school years, he'd been the target of racial bullying, receiving daily doses of punching, kicking, and pushing punctuated with the n-word, and no one came to his aid. Even as an adult, racist ideas followed him to a Cambridge street a dozen years ago while he walked at dusk and two white men yelled this word at him as they kicked him so many times in the head that when I found him at the hospital, I did not recognize him. A few years ago, he started experiencing panic attacks, and they seem to follow a pattern. They happen in the car when he's by himself, and immediately after another news report of a police shooting of an unarmed Black person pulled over for a routine traffic stop.

I thought about Alonso's mother in Kentucky, whose great-grandparents walked off plantations in the South, who drank from the "colored" water fountain in segregated Jim Crow-era Louisville, whose employer had lost a discrimination lawsuit for underpaying her for decades, who lost every penny of her retirement after entrusting it to a young white stockbroker who promised big returns on his tip, who rarely left her home to avoid the possibility of another white person humiliating her in everyday encounters.

Alonso had not personally contributed to this stereotype because when he was a kid, the only restaurant he ever ate at was McDonald's on Friday nights after his mother cashed her check. My friend's comment hung between us as the soft pretzel hardened and the beer cheese transformed into dried yellow paint. I was a coward in that moment and didn't argue with her observation, but instead gave in to my despair. I felt hopeless about our ability to overcome the obstacles in the conversation about race. Soon after, our friendship began to die. For months, I would walk by the river near dusk and allow myself to sob where no one would hear or see me. If we had still been friends, I would have shared my grief with her.

I don't believe that Becca is a bad person. Nor do I think that the women gossiping about my yellow children, or the school administrator, or the many people I hear casually drop insinuating comments about race would believe it if someone told them they harbored racist beliefs. But this is not about bad people. This is about a system of white supremacy that decent people, unaware of their power and privilege, enact and uphold. Even now, I reflexively want to protect my relationships with them at the expense of my own feelings. Like them, I'm also steeped in white supremacy. They too live in a world built on racism, colonialism, genocide, and other horrors. It is painful to look at, but that is preferable to pretending to ignore it.

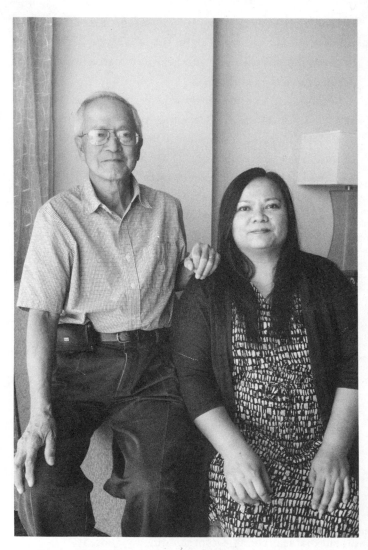

Grace and her father, Totoy, in fall 2018. Photo: Alonso Nichols.

16

The Small Red Fox

MY MOTHER COMPLAINS that since my father retired, he spends too much time watching YouTube videos of the Philippines. "What is he looking for?" she asks me. I don't tell her my theory: he's searching for what he's lost.

I've spent many hours sitting next to my father in a dark room watching a weekly news program from the Philippines called *I-Witness*, hosted by my friend Howie Severino. I've asked my father to watch Howie's show with me so that he can translate. Since returning from my time in the Philippines, I've missed my first country, especially the people, and watching the show reminds me that a place exists where being Filipino is normal.

I pause the video every few minutes so that my father can translate, often after he exclaims, "Oh no, no, no," or even swears.

"What is it, Dad?" I ask. "What's happening?"

In one episode, people are making coal by burning scrap wood. They're breathing smoke straight into their lungs, black dust coating their skin. The children will develop asthma; the adults, lung cancer. "This is Tondo, where I grew up," he says. "I didn't know they did this there."

In another episode, people are collecting discarded food from dumpsters and other trash bins. Fried chicken with only a few bites left on the bones, the last bit of pork adobo from a combo plate, expired frozen meat, slimy vegetables. First, they wash the food in boiling water. Then they season these second-hand scraps and eat them. Now they're spooning the leftover leftovers into clear plastic bags to sell. My father balances a piece of buttered toast on a paper towel, but he has stopped eating. Children the same age as his grandchildren dig through the refuse. An estimated 33 percent of Filipino children experience malnutrition or stunting according to 2015 data from the Food Nutrition and Research Institute. My father says, "Can you imagine? This is how hungry a person can be."

There's an episode that we don't finish about the extrajudicial killings, which number in the thousands. Since Philippine President Rodrigo Duterte was inaugurated in June 2016 and vowed to wage a war on drug users and pushers, in just over two years an estimated twelve to twenty thousand people, mostly urban poor suspected of being involved in the drug trade, have been killed by the Philippine National Police and unidentified gunmen. These astounding numbers include dozens of children who happened to be in the company of the adults who were shot, described by Duterte as "collateral damage" as well a few children targeted directly, including seventeen-year-old, unarmed Kian delos Santos, close circuit video footage of his execution death a counternarrative to the official one accusing him of shooting at officers during an anti-drug operation. At first, I don't understand what I'm seeing—the number of human-shaped plastic bags being loaded into the back of a garbage truck is beyond comprehension. And then a bag rips open and I recognize feet and legs, brown and hard, stacked like firewood.

Not every video is appalling. Through Howie, my father teaches me the history of the jeepney, describes how the Chabacano language evolved, and introduces me to the archipelago's remote beauty. He's pleased to see that his friends, also Filipino immigrants, are interviewed by Howie about the Aquino family's time in Massachusetts. Howie speaks with my father's *burkada*, his close friend group, and they tell stories I've heard before: what Ninoy's last night was like, how his goodbye felt final, and how, soon after that *despedida*, they received the call that he'd been assassinated on the tarmac at the Manila airport. Even after Ninoy's widow and then his son become presidents of the Philippines, they visit with the barkada when they make state visits to the U.S. The episode shows snapshots of the barkada having cookouts, going apple picking, and their favorite activity, playing mahjong. My father points to the younger version of his friends gleefully, but then he's suddenly quiet and grave. He pauses the video on his best friend, Tony, who moves mahjong tiles over the table. Almost every night for decades, my father played mahjong with Tony. Since his friend's death, my father has lost his desire to play.

Two of my father's brothers, Antonio and Cornelio, died within months of Tony. After each death, when I tried to comfort my father, he repeated what I'd heard him say all my life: "Gracie, that's the cycle of life. You start out going to baptisms and birthday parties, First Communions, debuts, graduations, and then weddings. But at a certain point, life is mostly funerals. Other people's funerals until it's time for yours."

For as long as I can remember, my father has prepared me for his death.

*

Immigration is a kind of death. You leave one life for another one with no guarantee of seeing your loved ones or home again. My cousin Jojo remembers that when his brother, Manong Ronnie, left for America, he thought their goodbye was forever. Flying to America was the same, in his mind, as dying and going to heaven. Before he left, Ronnie gave his brother a prayer card, something commonly given out at Catholic funerals. Much to Jojo's surprise, only weeks later, his visa came through and the brothers reunited. Jojo has carried this prayer card in his wallet ever since. Later, during Ronnie's funeral, Jojo reached into his back pocket, unfolded the card from his wallet, and waved it at us mourners.

My father is grateful that he spent his life in the U.S., but he also misses the Philippines. Perhaps watching the videos is his way to grieve for his first home, or to live vicariously. Maybe as he watches the scenes of daily life captured on CCTV camera he imagines himself back on those streets. Or maybe he just wants to hear his native tongue again after a lifetime of living in a second language. However, he complains that his understanding is limited—Filipinos use too many new words. "The population is really young," I say. "And language is a shifting, living thing. It changes as people discover a need to express new things. Isn't that fun?"

"But it's moving too fast for me," he says.

*

When he's not watching Philippine TV, my father is likely glued to a British nature show. For a while, he becomes singularly focused on a video of barnacle goslings leaving their nest. My siblings and I ask each other, "Has Dad shown you that barnacle gosling video yet? What's up with that?" We watch the five two-day-old goslings, the same number as my father's children, jump from their nest, high up on a barren cliff. Their parents and food wait at the bottom, but the goslings can't yet fly. From four hundred feet below, their parents call to them. "Come on. Jump already. Hurry!"

My father pauses the video. "There's nothing their parents can do. They can't help them," he explains. "They can only watch them fall."

I stare at him for a moment and wait for him to turn toward me. But he just resumes the video. The first chick jumps and my father holds his breath. The fluff of gray and white falls for an excruciatingly long time, almost thirty seconds. We wince when the chick bounces against rocks jutting from the cliff. We watch all five goslings leap, but only three get up and waddle toward their parents.

"Now watch this," my father says, wistfully. The camera follows a red fox running toward the goslings, who gather unaware at their parents' feet. They can't fly out of danger. I know he's viewed this moment dozens of times. Does he believe that if he watches it enough the video will end differently? "Even the cameraman can't help them, he's too far away. Hear how upset the cameraman is. He's so affected."

Suddenly, the fox arrives on the family scene, a shooting red arrow. "Gracie," my father says. "No one can stop the fox."

The parents squawk and spread their wings, but the fox is too fast. I am overcome with sadness. Who will call me Gracie once my father can't?

17

Foreign Bodies

AS AN OPHTHALMOLOGIST, my father has to deliver bad news fairly often. After thirty years of practicing medicine, he's learned to expect patients will resist and deny painful diagnoses, so he uses medical terminology—astigmatism, cataracts, macular degeneration—to give people something to hold on to.

I was photocopying insurance cards in his medical clinic when he told an elderly woman that she was legally blind. The woman was shocked. "But I can see fine," she insisted. She held her daughter's elbow, sobbing, as they trudged down the hallway to the waiting room. The woman couldn't see any less than when she had walked into my father's office.

Recently, he told me about a man who burst into tears when told that his child would need glasses. "But all the kids at school will make fun of him," the man said. "Maybe we can wait until he's a little older and bigger."

With calm, my father answered, "Your child's vision is blurry. He can't see the board at school. He can't see a car coming when he crosses the street."

*

I'm pressed against the picture window on the seventh floor at Massachusetts Eye and Ear. The Charles River shimmers, and for a weekday morning, there are a surprising number of sailboats gliding in figure eights. It's a beautiful day at the end of the summer. The kind of day that reminds us to hold on to it before it's gone, before the autumn forces us to retreat inside.

Ten adults crowd the hospital room, missing meetings and not returning phone calls or emails, so that we can sit around an empty bed. We're waiting for my two-year-old niece Naomi to return from emergency surgery to remove her right eye.

My mother sits in a plastic chair, counting the hours in rosaries, fingering each bead with a Hail Mary, again and again. My mother prays to her dead parents and siblings, begging them to whisper in God's ear and intercede on her behalf. Naomi's other grandparents, a preacher and his wife, whisper softly, an occasional "praise God" rising to my ears. Naomi's mother, my sister Ann, reads the latest *Harry Potter*, and Naomi's father Jorge talks on the phone, telling and retelling the story while we wait.

I notice Jorge is wearing the Superman T-shirt he wore on the day Naomi was born, the one inked with Naomi's newborn feet. It used to hang inside a box frame on the wall in his study, and I wonder about his decision to wear it. I imagine his loneliness and despair as he unhooks the frame from the wall, unpins the shirt, and pulls it over his head. These small actions are all he can do not to feel entirely helpless.

As soon as he heard the news, my brother Jet took a flight from Maui, traveling across the Pacific and then the continent. My other brother, Gerry, a first-year medical student at Boston University, skips his classes to sit with us. My husband Alonso waits here too. My sister Tessie, who is due to give birth any week now, calls us constantly from Los Angeles.

But there's a noticeable and puzzling absence: my father, the ophthalmologist. We act as if his absence proves the depth of his love for his granddaughter. He must love Naomi more than any of us, and that's why he's not here.

But I know the truth of why my father isn't here: he blames himself. If Naomi dies because he waited too long before voicing his suspicions about the subtle, almost imperceptible changes to her eye that he was the only one of us in a position to interpret—if Naomi dies because my father didn't say a word and the cancer eats her brain and spinal cord—I will blame him too.

*

Naomi's diagnosis took only seconds. The pediatric ophthalmologist just blinked into his ophthalmoscope before announcing, to everyone's shock, "Tumors. Looks like retinoblastoma."

And just as quickly, my father, who was in the exam room chatting with his former colleague, spun around and left the room without saying a word.

The team wanted to remove the eye immediately, but they couldn't schedule surgery until first thing the next day.

My father didn't speak much for the rest of the day, nor did he leave the car to attend the flurry of appointments with specialists before my niece's operation the next morning. I was in the car alone with him when he said miserably, "We could lose her."

"Not lose her," I countered. "Just her eye."

"Losing her eye," he said, "is the least of our worries."

*

While in training for his ophthalmology specialty thirty years ago at Philippine General Hospital, my father had witnessed enough cases of Rb to fear it. Some of the parents he met had read the mysterious white glow from their toddlers' eyes as a sign that their child was special, embodied with powers to divine the future or bring the family luck.

"Stupid," my father said. He watched their children die.

Once Naomi was diagnosed, Ann recalled moments in the past months where she saw a strange reflection from the night light in Naomi's right eye, like the glow of a cat's eye. But the conditions had to be just right, and Ann didn't see it all the time, so it didn't alarm her.

As the first grandchild in our family, Naomi was the most photographed child in our history. That night after hearing about Naomi's diagnosis, my father studied hundreds of photos of her. "I didn't see it," he said. "How could I not see it?"

Every month since Naomi's birth, Ann has posed Naomi with a stuffed Tigger and posted these photos to her baby blog. The baby blog meticulously documents "firsts" in Naomi's life, which, considering she's just turned two, is almost everything. But the last picture, instead of merely celebrating her growth, showed Naomi's tumor. In the flash photography, the tumor in her right eye was obvious, unmistakable. Instead of normal red eye reflex, Naomi's right eye was an opaque pearl. In a handful of other photos from the past four months, there were hints of the white spot in her eye, slight irregularities. There it was while Naomi blew out two birthday candles, while she sat with my father watching television after a summer cookout, while she posed indoors next to Clifford the Big Red Dog on an excursion to Boston's Children's Museum.

But clues are not enough. An eye exam in a darkened room with an ophthalmoscope would have caught the gooey tumors as they started to gather and grow. Instead, for months, the cancer cells on her retina spread until they detached her retina, blinding her in that eye, and none of us knew.

*

We didn't know how much we needed Naomi until she came into our lives. When she was a year old, Ann and my brother-in-law Jorge moved in with my parents to save money for a house. My parents were delighted. For almost a decade after their five children had left the nest, their house had been empty. There were rooms, full of our old clothes, that my parents didn't enter anymore. The first time I visited my parents' house after Naomi moved in, I walked up the green carpeted stairs and found one fuzzy pink sock, then a plush rattle. I heard laughter. Effusive. Explosive. Joyous. It had been so long.

Naomi performs daily miracles we can't live without: She's thrown open the bulkhead door in the cellar where my father hoards his love. She shines herself at us and says, "I love you."

During that first year at my parents' house, one day a week Naomi was mine. I would leave my apartment before 7 a.m. so I could be the first person to greet Naomi when she awoke; it was me who performed the morning rituals of diaper change, warm milk bottle, and snuggling. My name was one of her first words, and her parents taught her to add the Filipino word for aunt, "tita." As her vocabulary grew, I was Tee Grace, then Tee Tah Grace; and then she sang my name into a birdcall like the northern bobwhite, Tee Ta Grace.

We attended a Mommy and Me-type music class together, and I pretended to be her mommy. The first time I brought her there she was so anxious that she vomited. The next couple of classes she sat on my lap and held my arms around her like a scarf as she watched the other children dance and sing. Then one day, she jumped out of my lap as soon as the teacher began to play the guitar, and before I knew it, Naomi was leading the toddler mosh pit.

That year with Naomi held some of the happiest moments of my life. We threw handfuls of cereal onto the living room floor and let her dog Gordie, a 170-pound presa canario, clean it up. We emptied a container of baby powder in her bedroom when she missed the snow. We tossed pizza dough into the air and cracked eggs against the counter and spooned soil with ice cream scoops into seedling trays on the coffee table. After our day together, I'd feed her and bathe her. I'd rock her on my belly and tell her a story, then continue retelling it until Naomi stopped saying, again, again, again.

*

As the daughter of an ophthalmologist, I was constantly aware of my eyes. The world I knew was riddled with dangers. My father prohibited us from throwing snowballs or eating lollipops or filling out crossword puzzles in the car or letting the dog lick our face. I learned to respect the raw power of drinking straws, metal clothes hangers, baseballs, pencils, and tree branches.

When I started working for my father at age eight, earning a few pennies for each medical chart I completed by pasting in multicolored chart numbers, he told me about foreign bodies. "Foreign bodies—dust, metal shavings, wood chips," he explained, "prevent people from seeing. Sometimes they make your eye infected, and sometimes they can make you blind."

I imagined miniature men in ethnic costumes kicking as my father plucked them from the whites of his patients' eyes.

My father saved up stories from the hospital and transformed them into directives: Never let a parrot sit on your shoulder, I don't care how well you think you know him. (One of his patients liked to feed her parrot almonds that she balanced on her lips, until the parrot mistook her eye for an almond.) Don't carry pencils, sharpened end up, in your shirt pocket. Watch out for corners on bookshelves and tabletops, or better yet, only buy furniture with rounded edges. Avoid long-stemmed roses, popsicles, high heel shoes, and hardcover books. No jumping on the bed, look what happened to your brother.

My brother Jet was almost two when he fell from the bed, hitting his eye on the corner of the wooden headboard and falling to the floor. My father carried Jet through the emergency room of his hospital, past the waiting room and nurses' station. He sat my screaming brother on a bed and pulled the yellow curtain around them. My father didn't trust the resident on call, didn't trust anyone but himself to hold the sharp points of the syringe, the threaded needle, and surgical scissors close to Jet's eye. My mother helped hold my brother down. My father sobbed as he sewed the stitches, but his hand was steady and careful. He understood how a scarred and disfigured eye could impact his son's future. The pink scar drawn underneath Jet's left eyebrow is a faded testament to close calls and my father's expert hands.

But now, with Naomi's diagnosis, I feel betrayed. I want to tell him, *You taught me to be afraid of pens and lollipops and snowballs and rose bushes and everything else in the world when all this time the danger was inside of us.*

*

When we tell the story of Naomi's cancer, my father comes out the hero. It was he who first noticed that Naomi's right eye was slightly misaligned. During the Easter holidays, I heard him murmuring about strabismus, or lazy eye, and a month later he began to share his suspicions regularly to any of us who would listen. At a Mother's Day meal, my cousin Rod, also a physician, admitted that he thought Naomi was going cross-eyed.

But despite all the talk, no one was alarmed. We didn't want to consider that she might be imperfect; we didn't think her misaligned eyes could threaten anything but her looks. Silent alarms were firing in my father's head, but he didn't voice his fears.

Tessie was married that Memorial Day weekend, and all through the festivities my father placed one hand, then the other, in front of Naomi's eyes. He would sneak his hand around from behind and try to cover Naomi's eye, but she was a toddler. She would get annoyed and swat it away.

"Leave her alone," I said. "She doesn't like that."

Months later, after Naomi's cancer was diagnosed, my father, in a story he can't stop telling, a story that implicates him again and again, tells me that he'd been trying to check Naomi's visual field. "But she saw my hand," he says. "She saw it."

I understand what he needs. Forgiveness, relief from culpability. "You couldn't have known," I said. And it's true. Without a proper exam with the right instruments, he couldn't have. But I wish he had said, "I doubt it's anything serious, but I've noticed Naomi's right eye is wandering to the side. It's my professional recommendation that you take her to a doctor."

*

The irony is that my father, the ophthalmologist, doesn't believe in going to the doctor. His medicine cabinet is full of prescriptions he's written for himself—antibiotics for sore throats and topical creams for his eczema. (At least, he thinks it's eczema; he's never been to a dermatologist to find out for sure.) He has health insurance, and plenty of his physician friends would see him for free—that's not the problem. The problem is that he understands far too well how disease waits for everybody, and part of him still believes that not acknowledging a problem will make it go away.

My father's not unusual among his friends: cardiologists who smoke and drink, psychiatrists and gynecologists who fall asleep in the middle of a booze-filled weekend mahjong binge. They believe their status and training as doctors makes them unsusceptible to the body's limits. One colleague, who had two children under the age of six, was covered in bruises and so fatigued that she was crawling up the stairs. The doctors confirmed what she already knew—leukemia—and she was dead in three months. By the time another friend, a psychiatrist, was diagnosed with lung cancer, the only option was palliative care, a pain-free dream he slipped into for a several weeks, and then he was gone. Like them, my doctor father neglects his body, and I have inherited his self-destructive habits: smoking, over- and undereating, over- and underexercising, sitting so still my legs fall asleep, holding my urine until I'm in pain.

*

By summer, all five of my brothers and sisters, their significant others, my parents, and everyone else in my niece's life weighed in with their opinions: Does she or does she not have a lazy eye?

"Call it amblyopia," I said. "Lazy is so judgmental."

Many times, we'd poked fun at people with misaligned eyes: the popcorn vendor at the cinema, the clerks at the town library, the odd colleague with poor social skills. We laughed, "Which eye do we look at when we're talking to him?" Children are so cruel; adults, even crueler.

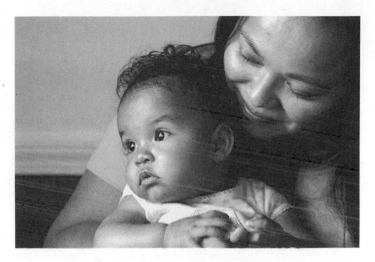

Grace and her niece Naomi a year before Naomi is diagnosed with eye cancer. Photo: Alonso Nichols.

In early July, my friend revealed that she had surgery as a toddler to correct her wandering eye. Now her eyes are perfectly aligned, and this information gave me courage to insist. I told my sister, "Get some medical advice about Naomi's eye from an ophthalmologist who isn't also her grandfather."

I was overstepping a line. Never interfere between parent and child. It's none of my business; her parents know what's best for her. But for Naomi, I found new courage.

Almost five months had passed from when the question began to form in my father's mind. The tumors had grown very quickly, and in that time Naomi's eye became blind. There's no guarantee doctors could have saved the eye even if they'd found the cancer early, and in a way, finding the cancer at its final stage was a blessing. Now there was no choice but to remove the eye. Maybe if it had been caught earlier, they would have been tempted to save it through radiation or other treatments that can be painful and disfiguring. If the Rb cells had been allowed to escape and tumors were found outside of the eye, Naomi's survival rate would have dropped to less than ten percent.

*

On the morning before Naomi's surgery, after Ann and Jorge dress Naomi in the surgical gown, they take a last family photo with Naomi's right eye. Naomi wears a yellow gown that opens in the back, and thick hospital socks with rough treads on the feet. Her thick curls aren't brushed, and she's crying.

After surgery, they will perform scans and biopsies and spinal taps and mine bone marrow. In order to have easy access to Naomi's vascular system, they hide a plastic port, like a piece of uncooked ziti, under the skin next to her left nipple. They need this easy entrance to her body to infuse her with chemo and test her blood. Her baby-smooth skin is bruised from the needles and raw from bandage adhesive.

After surgery, Naomi does not speak or even cry. Ann lies on the bed and Naomi settles underneath her mother's breasts as if she's an enraged squatter trying to move back inside the only home where she ever felt safe. If anyone tries to kiss or touch Naomi or if Ann readjusts her position, Naomi shrieks like a wild animal. She has white bandages over her right eye, protruding like a fist.

Immediately after surgery, we discover that they've found no sign of cancer in the other eye, and that on first glance, there are no obvious signs of spreading. All good news.

As we wait for Naomi's anesthesia to wear off, we sit together in the hospital room and wait. We look out the window so we don't have to look at each other. We eat soup and drink coffee. We make excuses about why my father, the ophthalmologist, isn't here for his granddaughter's eye surgery. We understand that like all of us, he's doing the best he can.

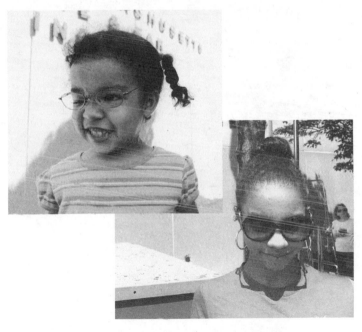

Grace's niece Naomi (above) the day after enucleation surgery to remove the eye with cancer and (below) at the same spot more than a decade later.

POSITIVE FOR A DELETERIOUS MUTATION

Test Performed	Result	Interpretation
Q1538X *BRCA1*	Q1538X	Deleterious

This test is designed to detect the specific mutation(s) or variant(s) indicated above.

The results of this analysis are consistent with the germline BRCA1 mutation Q1538X, resulting in premature truncation of the BRCA1 protein at amino acid position 1538. Although the exact risk of breast and ovarian cancer conferred by this specific mutation has not been determined, studies in high-risk families indicate that deleterious mutations in BRCA1 may confer as much as an 87% risk of breast cancer and a 44% risk of ovarian cancer by age 70 in women (Lancet 343:692-695, 1994). Mutations in BRCA1 have been reported to confer a 20% risk of a second breast cancer within five years of the first (Lancet 351:316-321, 1998), as well as a ten-fold increase in the risk of subsequent ovarian cancer (J Clin Oncol 16:2417-2425, 1998). This mutation may also confer an increased (albeit low) risk of male breast cancer (Am J Hum Genet 62:676-689, 1998), as well as some other cancers. Each first degree relative of this individual has a one-in-two chance of having this mutation. Family members can be tested for this specific mutation with a single site analysis.

Test results showing that Grace is a carrier of the BRCA1 gene mutation, which confers a high lifetime risk of breast and ovarian cancers.

18

Carriers

WHEN I WAS FIFTEEN, my maternal grandmother Mama Lola threatened to cut her breasts off with a steak knife. She was visiting from the Philippines and had been constantly bickering with my mother since she'd arrived. One day, the fight exploded, leading to Mama Lola standing in the kitchen, the top of her housedress unbuttoned, with a steak knife pressed against the flat spot between her long, deflated breasts.

"I fed you from these mammary glands. I sacrificed everything for my nine children, and this is how you talk to me?" she said.

My mother looked up briefly, sighed, and went back to wiping rice from placemats. "Enough, Ma," my mother sighed. She brought a stack of the lunch dishes to the kitchen sink.

Mama Lola followed like a nipping puppy and said, "I will cut these off. They are useless now. Like me."

My mother dropped the dishes noisily into the sink and, in a voice I've never heard her use since, screamed, "Get out of here!"

By this point in her life, my mother was tired of grandparents. She had been in America long enough to form an identity that was separate from her mother. She found her voice and it was angry. Filial piety was cast aside; my mother would choose her children's well-being over anyone else's feelings again and again. These were the years my mother permed her hair, and even her curls seemed to express her rage. When relatives from the Philippines, as a way of greeting me after a long absence, would exclaim how fat I was, my mother scolded them that we didn't comment on people's bodies in the States. The meek, loyal, respectful version of Norma was gone.

I don't know if my mother meant for my grandmother to leave, or us, her five children, but Tessie and I quickly gathered the younger children and went to the movies.

We returned later that night and my grandmother was gone. I visited with her a few times in the Philippines before she died, but she was never allowed in our house again. I have often wondered why my grandmother chose her breasts as the body part to threaten to slice off. Why not poke out an eye or chop off a hand? Or maybe an ear like Van Gogh?

*

During those years, my mother Norma was in constant motion, cleaning, shopping, cooking, driving, and managing everyone else's lives. Back in the Philippines, there were people who did these things for her. Every little thing. She grew up attending the country's most elite private schools accompanied by her yaya, who tied her shoes, carried her book bag, and waited outside her classroom until it was time to give Norma her lunch. After school, Norma sent an errand boy to the park, about a mile walk away, to fetch her a small cone of peanuts fried with thin slices of garlic. It would have been more efficient for him to buy a bag that would last the week, but Norma preferred her snack freshly fried and warm.

My mother told this story recently to her nine-year old grandson Evan. "The boy who fetched me warm peanuts every day was your age," she said. "He kind of looked like you."

"Shouldn't he have been in school?" I asked.

My mother said that her parents sent the younger household helpers to school, even college courses.

"Really?" I asked, skeptically. "Why would they do that?"

My mother said that her family treated their helpers differently than most other families in her class—not the wealthiest, old-money class, but in the higher income bracket for sure. Her ancestors had been landowners and grew sugar and rice, but this wealth was largely gone by her generation. Her father worked for a living as a police detective and her mother was a teacher, but they received some financial help from his elderly great-aunts in the province that elevated their class status.

"Evan," I said. "When your grandmother was your age, she was a spoiled, rich brat."

She had a hard time when she first came to the States. "I cried every day," she said. "It was hell." She had never washed a dish or piece of clothing before. She did not know about laundry machines and, for the first few months, washed our family's clothes in a bucket. My father bought rope to hang a line through the living room to dry the clothes.

"My hands were cut up from scrubbing your clothes so hard," she said. "My knees and shoulders have never recovered because after you went to sleep, I would get on my hands and knees and scrub the floors clean."

"Why didn't anyone tell you about washing machines and dryers?" I asked. "Didn't you have friends?"

"I knew nothing," she said. My father taught her, the same way he taught all of us children, how to make rice the Filipino way, and how to wash the rice and measure the water by swirling the grains until they were level and marking the spot with your thumb. She practiced recipes from cookbooks and eventually made friends with other Filipinas who shared their recipes. "I was miserable and didn't know how to do anything domestic, but there was something in me that wanted to fight," she said. "I wanted to prove that I could make it on my own in the States."

When we were born, my mother hired one yaya each for my sister Tessie and me. Their only job was to care for us. Others—the *lavandera*, the driver, the houseboy, the cook— performed the many household chores. But in America, my mother noticed the other women doing it all themselves. She was determined to become like them. She made friends with a neighbor, Sue, who introduced her to other women. They drank tea in the afternoons and took classes together in ceramics, holiday crafts, and aerobics. My mother always returned from her outings re-energized and refreshed. One day she came back with her hair cut pixie short, like 1980s rockers Pat Benatar and Joan Jett, and at first I didn't recognize her. She was buoyant and hopeful. She looked like a woman who satisfied her own desires first, not someone who was disappointed in herself and resentful for giving up her career as a doctor to serve her husband and children.

As we grew up and needed her less, my mother was ambitious. She thought she might try to be a doctor again. After she cut her hair, she signed up to study for the exam for foreign medical graduates. I remember her excitement and how for a season, she disappeared in the afternoons to study. I imagine Norma driving the hour to the test prep center and settling into a carrel with her materials, reviving her knowledge from two decades earlier. See how she concentrates with pencil in hand and recalls what had been pushed to the back of her mind by diapers, immigration, and recipes from women's magazines? But one afternoon, she realizes how tired she is from trying to have it all, and instead of turning into the test center, she exits at the mall. She talks to sales people who are happy to see her, a doctor's wife flush with cash, until it's time to go home. She feels the thrill of getting away with something. And the next day, Norma goes to see a movie, and the next, she eats lunch in a restaurant by herself for the first time, staring out the window, losing track of time, but finding the sound of her voice. It says, "Too late." The next day, she gets in the car, intent on driving to the test prep center. Norma circles the parking lot, looking for the best spot, but discouraged, she finds herself turning back onto the highway toward home.

We noticed our mother was back at home in the afternoons, but we knew not to ask why.

*

I think of my thirties as the cancer years. First my niece Naomi, then my older sister Tessie, then me, and finally my younger sister Ann were forced to contend with cancer as a threat and a reality.

My father passed down the faulty gene through his mother, Inang. My grandmother was a strong and healthy woman, a survivor. My aunt Abigail tells a story about how Inang, visibly pregnant, was at the market with her one day during World War II when Japanese soldiers showed up, looking for the local men. In the commotion and fear, my Inang slid under a table and hid Abigail under her dress, between her legs.

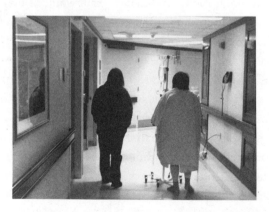

Grace (left) walks her sister Ann down the hallway after Ann's preventive mastectomy. Photo: Alonso Nichols.

Since my father is a known carrier, his offspring have a 50-50 chance of carrying the gene. Affected offspring in turn have a 50-50 chance of passing it on to their children.

Ms. Chan, my genetic counselor, happened to work in the same medical complex as the hospital room where my sister Tessie was recovering from a bilateral mastectomy. She had endured chemo, radiation, and now surgery. I promised Tessie that I would visit her after my appointment with the genetic counselor. "Good luck," she said weakly. Her bare head was covered with a cap, her skin gray. She looked almost dead.

"I have a really good feeling," I told her. "No worries."

I could tell from the way my genetic counselor's voice sounded on the phone that my results were going to be negative. In other words, positive, something to celebrate.

I sat at the small table with Ms. Chan, smiling. Alonso was next to me smiling, too. I told him that morning that he didn't need to come with me and miss work. I was going to get good news. In my mind, I had already endured enough bad things for one lifetime. The rest would be icing.

Ms. Chan pushed a piece of paper at me. "So here are your results," she said flatly. "You're positive for the gene."

I surprised myself by bursting into tears.

"I'm so sorry," she said. "I hate this fucking gene."

I returned to my sister's hospital room after I got the news. Tessie tried to smile at me, but instead, grimaced in pain. "I am just so happy," she said. "That you don't have to go through what I've gone through. You can prevent this."

Now she says I'm lucky. I don't have to live in fear that rogue cancer cells are hiding out in my bones or brain, waiting to show up one day to ruin my life. Tessie can't talk about the chemotherapy, but I remember her complaining about how the oncology nurse would dress in a space suit and thick gloves to protect herself from the bright red liquid that she inserted directly into her vein. Even now, if my sister—my tough sister who fiercely fought off all sorts of attacks as an immigrant Asian girl—gets a simple flu shot or a finger prick, she can't help crying.

With hereditary breast and ovarian cancer, each affected generation shows earlier ages of diagnosis. My grandmother Inang died of breast cancer two years after being diagnosed at age eighty-two. The next generation, my aunts, were diagnosed with breast and ovarian cancer in their fifties and sixties. And the next generation, my cousins and sister, were in their thirties and forties when they were diagnosed with breast cancer.

Tessie had just had a baby and thought the lump was a clogged milk duct. Her doctors thought the lump was a clogged milk duct too. The tumor grew over a period of months, unchecked, and spread to her lymph nodes. When I saw my sister before her first treatment, it was a warm day and she wore a thin shirt. I could see the tumor bulging slightly from her right breast as she held her baby in her arms. To cheer her up during treatment, I gave her a comic book, *Cancer Made Me a Shallower Person: A Memoir in Comics*, by Miriam Engelberg. We laughed together while reading it.

A few months later, when the author died from complications due to breast cancer, I didn't tell my sister.

*

Instead of amputating my breasts, people advised, I could eat better and exercise more. "Lose weight," they said. I was told I should hold off on the preventive surgeries—a cure for cancer might be only a few years away. Besides, why worry about breast cancer when I could get hit by a bus or die in a car accident? Women who receive a breast cancer diagnosis choose lumpectomies and radiation, so why would I consider an action so drastic as to remove my breasts?

It didn't sway critics when I informed them that hereditary breast cancer meant my lifetime risk was up to 87 percent from the standard 13 percent; and for ovarian cancer, between 10 and 60 percent up from the standard 1.5 percent risk. Yet I had trouble understanding what those numbers meant. I finally acted when I glimpsed my future, and saw misery. As my friend Gilmore said, "If someone is forcing you to eat a shit sandwich, you may as well take a small bite."

After months of research, surveillance tests, and conversations, I agreed to a preventive mastectomy scheduled for the day after my fall classes ended. In the days before the surgery, I stopped in front of the bathroom mirror after showering to memorize my breasts. In the sleepless nights before the surgery, I held my breasts in my hands. I thought of how the first buds appeared through my electric-blue dance costume at age eleven; how water felt like velvet when I swam topless with my girlfriends in the summer.

The morning of my surgery, my parents drove from an hour away to pick me up at my apartment. I lived just eight minutes from the hospital. I took an Ativan as soon as I woke up, and by the time I got in the car with my parents, I was in a great mood. I made them laugh as we drove over the Zakim bridge.

My father dropped us off at Massachusetts General and kissed me on the cheek, a rare gesture. My parents bickered in Tagalog. They did this because they didn't want us to know they were fighting, but you didn't have to comprehend the words to understand the tone. "Aren't you staying with us?" my mother asked.

"I have patients," he said.

"Not for a few more hours," she insisted.

My father is brave in many ways. And in others, he is so terrified he can barely function, paralyzed by his feelings. He drove an hour back to his ophthalmology office, reclined in a yellow leather chair in one of his exam rooms, and fell asleep until the secretaries arrived.

I changed and lay down on a gurney. The nurse pulled a sheet over me. She asked if I want my visitors to wait with me. While I waited for Alonso and my mother, a woman in a white coat asked if she could start an IV. "I'm just going to put something in to relax you, you might feel dizzy," she said. I nodded. The woman crouched, slid a syringe from her pocket, and pushed the liquid into my hand.

A moment later, I woke up shivering cold and desperate to pee. My voice was so soft it didn't reach the nurses working around me. I was afraid I might wet the bed. "I just need the toilet one more time before the surgery," I said.

"You're all done," the nurse said. "You did great. We're going to take you up to your room in just a minute."

"But when will I have the surgery?" I asked.

And then I looked down at my chest and saw the bloody drains pinned to my gown and the white of the surgical bra strapped around me. I tried to sit up, but I was too sore. My body was a pain cage. In that moment, I lost my fear of death. About six hours had gone in a blink of an eye. It was that easy to be and not to be.

*

I'd opted for a simple subcutaneous mastectomy with immediate reconstruction; I was on the operating table for about six hours. I didn't recognize myself in those intensely painful first days after the surgery—I floated alone despite all the good wishes, flowers, and cards. Tessie assured me that I would heal a little more every day. She told me to look for signs, even if they were barely perceptible, that I was getting better.

When I finally mustered the nerve to look at myself, undressing for my first post-surgery shower, I stood in front of the mirror and bawled. Under the clear tape covering the incision, where my nipples used to be, a black line was drawn over each breast in dried blood. The implant was smaller than my breasts had been. Without nipples, my breasts looked like a pair of seamed socks pulled over closed fists, or two tight mouths with lips wrapped around teeth.

My mother knocked softly on my bedroom door. She ran the shower and would help me bathe. "Ready?" she asked.

Throughout my recovery, my mother rallied. She lined up my pills in the morning and cooked all my favorite food, even though I had no appetite. When I am on my deathbed, my mother is the one I would want to nurse me, but she's already told me that she wants to die before her children.

"Hold on," I whined. I was surprised by how annoyed my voice sounded, like an exasperated teenager getting ready for a dance.

On my left side, I had a concave area near my pectoralis major. I pushed three fingers into the slope, pressing against my sternum, my fingertips sinking into the skin until they stopped against muscle and bone. I hadn't expected this hollowing out of my chest, and I was horrified by the concavity, this bowl scraped clean.

Suddenly, I was overwhelmed with regret: I wanted my breasts back.

*

Eight months after the surgery, I went in for the follow-up. I didn't smile and answered my doctor's questions in the flattest tone possible. My breast surgeon was a trim woman with short brown hair. She was intelligent, highly skilled, warm, and thoughtful, but after the mastectomy, I was angry at her for taking what was mine. For months, I had canceled follow-up appointments and ignored phone calls from her office to come in. I saw my plastic surgeon, the person who reconstructed me, happily, but I did not want to see the person who removed my breasts.

I opened the gown and turned my head to study the floor tiles as my doctor's fingers touched my skin. I knew she was looking at my scars: the lines under my right arm where lymph nodes were removed; two five-inch scars over my breast mounds; on both sides of my ribcage, scars the size of pencil erasers healed over the holes where plastic drains snaked out of my body; two raised scars like permanent mosquito bites on my right breast where a long needle cored into my tissue for biopsies.

"Looks good," my doctor said.

When I finally spoke, I asked, "So what did you do with them? My breasts. Where are they?"

My doctor explained that they were weighed, some samples were preserved in paraffin for examination by pathology, and the rest was discarded.

*

Tessie was right, as usual. I got better. I found community in the early days of an online bulletin board led by Sue Friedman, a former veterinarian who became the founder and executive director of an organization called FORCE: Facing Our Risk of Cancer. Sue awarded me a scholarship to attend their annual conference that focuses on people who are affected by hereditary cancer or a genetic mutation associated with an increased risk of cancer. I learned the term "previvors"—those who haven't yet developed cancer, but who carry a predisposition. I met people who'd given up more vital body parts than I had—their colon, their uterus—to reduce their cancer risk.

A few years ago, I attended a FORCE conference with Ann and my cousin Marie, who both have the BRCA1 mutation and were considering preventive mastectomies, and dragged them to an evening event where women were invited to show each other their post-operative chests and talk about their recovery processes in a more relaxed atmosphere. At some point, after some wine, I surprised myself by taking off my shirt at the crowded party. No one would ever mistake what I have now for what I had before the mastectomy, but I wasn't ashamed to show the reality of my body. I did not hide the failed nipples that my plastic surgeon tried to make in her office one afternoon, tattooing a dark circle over my mastectomy scar, then slicing the skin and stitching the edges into a burgundy top hat. I was impressed with her technique; she made them pretty. I didn't know I cared about having nipples until I saw myself in the doctor's mirror. Something inside me unclenched. From a distance, I almost looked like myself again. Unfortunately, the nipples didn't take and now there were brown smudges where the top hats had been, but I wasn't ashamed. I allowed the curious women to feel the size and weight of my breasts, to trace where my implant was attached to muscle.

It's been several years since my surgery, and I hardly ever think about my lost breasts. I'm grateful for my "breast mounds"—a fair trade for peace of mind and the opportunity to escape breast cancer.

*

Every now and then my father will bring up my mastectomy. Perhaps he feels guilty for being the one who passed on the genetic mutation. Some of our relatives have died too young, from cancer. "You did the right thing," he always says. "I know it was hard. But you are still alive."

After my mastectomy, I didn't go running for almost two years. The first time, I wore two sports bras and crossed my arms against my chest, cupping each breast in a hand. I was terrified that running would cause my silicone implants to burst from my skin. I imagined them bouncing and rolling on the track in front of me. I saw myself stooping to collect the slippery implants, and quickly dusting off the black pebbles from the track before anyone saw.

*

My life went in a different and unexpected direction after I received the test results confirming that I was a carrier for the BRCA1 gene mutation. I felt I had entered a room where the ceiling was slowly but surely lowering toward my head. I had some unknown amount of time—months, maybe years—to make some hard decisions about how to leave that room. For several years, my life spun around the centripetal force of two questions. Should we have biological children? And, had I put off answering the first question for so long that now I already had cancer? I read an article about a woman younger than I was with the same gene mutation. She thought she might have another child and waited to have the surgery, but in the meantime, she developed ovarian cancer and died.

What to do with the parts of my body that would likely develop cancer put pressure on an already time-sensitive and contentious issue between my husband and me: whether to have children. In short, I wanted them, and he didn't. Of course, it's more complicated and nuanced than that. Sometimes I didn't, and most of the time Alonso wasn't sure. Early on in our relationship, I thought this had been decided. We seemed to share the same dream: no more than three children. We spent many hours talking about if we wanted to be parents and how we would manage if we did. At times, I swung toward wanting children, but then decided it would be too hard.

In the time it takes to raise a baby to adulthood, we talked and waited for our lives to get better. We hesitated so long that we were almost too old, and only the question remained: Yes or no?

We had a very long engagement as we worked to finish graduate school, establish our careers, pay off tuition, and save money to own a home. The time came when we had saved enough to host our own small wedding. We discussed whether we should try and have a child. I took prenatal vitamins to prepare my body.

*

Even though I was still angry about the unfolding child sexual abuse in the church, I wanted the sacrament of marriage in the Catholic Church. We met with the priest who would celebrate the nuptial mass. He read through a list of questions and then asked, "Would you accept children if they came into your marriage?"

I looked over at Alonso and saw that he was nodding. I felt a spark of hope and joy. A few months later, Alonso and I attended a weekend at a marriage preparation course, a requirement to be married in the Catholic Church. The course was held in an overheated church basement next to Boston Common. We listened to presentations, filled out worksheets, and did communication exercises. At the seminar on modern life and real-world Catholicism, I raised my hand to ask a question about the Church's stance on terminating an early pregnancy if it was discovered that the fetus had a genetic abnormality. By then, I was of the age that a pregnancy would have been categorized as geriatric, and I didn't think I had the resources, emotional and financial, to care for a child with severe disabilities. I also wondered what the Church stance was on reproductive medicine. A few people had told me that if we went the fertility clinic route, we should select for fetuses that did not carry the BRCA1 gene mutation via pre-implantation genetic diagnosis. It was all so mind-blowing, these god-like decisions we had the power to make now that new technologies existed in reproductive medicine to select offspring without the mutation. I was surprised and relieved by the answer I got from Catholic leaders that day. The priest assured us that whatever we decided was best for us as a couple was what we should do.

Later that afternoon, in a large circle with fifty other betrothed, Alonso and I stood back to back, sweating through our shirts. The priest leading the exercise asked questions about housework preferences (dishes for me and laundry for him), finances (both of us needed to generate income), and other issues, and we recorded our answers onto index cards. We turned to face each other and show our answers. It was a lighthearted exercise and couples laughed as they read their mate's card. Then, the priest asked how many children we wanted. Alonso and I revealed our cards.

I had written ">1" to Alonso's "0."

Alonso read my card and immediately whipped a pen out of his pocket. He crossed off "0," replacing it with "~1."

My stomach flipped with hope. The switch had flipped. If Alonso wanted approximately one child, then perhaps we could compromise on my desire to have a number greater than one. A single child would still make me a mother.

*

Some months later after our wedding, we honeymooned in the Philippines. It was a brief trip, just ten days, and Alonso's first time in Asia. My relatives pestered us about when we would start our family. "Don't wait too long," they said.

Every time they asked, my face would pink up even more in the tropical heat. "We're not quite ready," I said. I was in my thirties, which I'm sure seemed ancient to my cousins in the Philippines who had started families in their early twenties.

"What are you waiting for?" they asked.

I wanted to pay off my student loans; I wanted to publish a book; I wanted to buy a home.

My relatives were baffled. "Okay, but what do any of these things have to do with starting a family?" Besides, they told me, it wasn't up to us. God would either grant us a child or not. We just needed to open ourselves to the opportunity to receive the gift. "At least have one," they said, as if they were presenting me with a plate of sweets that I kept politely refusing.

One tita, who I had not seen in many years, introduced herself to my husband and once the small talk was over, rubbed my belly, feeling all the contours from top to bottom, hip to hip. I was speechless.

"What's going on inside here?" she asked.

"Nothing," I said. "I overeat sometimes."

"How many kids do you have?" she asked.

"Zero," I said too loudly.

She wrinkled her nose as if I had just burped in her face. I could guess what she was thinking. *How could you, a married couple, perfectly healthy, and gainfully employed, not bring new souls into this world?* She finally took her hand off of my belly, which had only found fat in its search for a kicking fetus, and shook her finger at my husband. "They say that a wife looks like this," her eyes went to the part of my body that I try to hide with loose shirts and draped sweaters, "to remind you of what she really wants. It's okay, I will pray for you. But you need to try harder to put a baby in there."

*

We returned home from our honeymoon, and I continued my screening protocol for ovarian cancer. My doctor didn't want to pressure me to remove my ovaries, but I could tell that she thought I should get them taken out sooner rather than later. Which would mean the end of babies.

Even though it was recommended that I have the oophorectomy at age thirty-five, I wanted to wait at least a year after the mastectomy I had that year. As I turned thirty-six and then thirty-seven, my cancer surgeon reminded me that the benefit of knowing my genetic predisposition was to prevent ovarian cancer. There was a preventive surgery, a bilateral salpingo-oophorectomy—a surgical procedure that would excise both my ovaries and fallopian tubes—that would significantly reduce my risk of developing ovarian cancer. I was counseled to have this surgery when I reached the age of forty (some doctors say age thirty-five) or had completed childbearing, whichever came sooner. Chemoprevention and surveillance were also options, but surgery was the best tool to manage ovarian cancer risk: the lifetime risks of ovarian cancer in the general population is 1.5 percent, but women with BRCA mutations have up to a 60 percent lifetime risk and tend to develop ovarian cancer at a younger age.

*

Time was running out. My doctor prescribed prenatal vitamins in case we changed our minds and I wanted to get pregnant before my next screening appointment. But my husband still wasn't sure. For years, this longing clouded my life. I already was so fortunate and privileged. I had a lot of what I wanted out of life—love, friends, travel, meaningful work. I should not be asking for more. In fact, I thought I would be punished for it. Part of me knew this made no sense, but I had been shaped by the idea that anything bad that had happened in my life had been my own fault. Maybe I would die in childbirth.

For years, when I spotted a multiracial child that could be ours, of African American and Asian ancestry, I would yearn hard. Discreetly, I'd point the child out to Alonso in the hopes that he would recognize these future unborn children and want them, too. Early in our dating life, he would play the game and imagine what our children would look like, half Filipino and half Black, half him, half me. But as time went on, he seemed less interested and I became more so.

A consolation and source of comfort in not having my own children yet was my relationship with my nieces and nephews. They all lived within an easy drive from me and I would spend at least one day a week with some configuration of them. When they were toddlers, they would hear me come up the stairs and gather behind the baby gate, rattling it and calling, *Teetah! Teetah!* It was what I looked forward to in my grind as a freelancer and adjunct. No matter how tired I was, on a day that I was going to spend with them, I hopped right out of bed and braved the morning traffic through Boston joyfully.

But one by one, my siblings moved their young families away. I was devastated, but silent. These children might be the closest I'd get to parenthood, but what rights did I have as their aunt? All I could do was tell them I'd miss them and wish them well.

Alonso and I talked about other routes to parenthood—adoption and gestational surrogates—so that I could have the oophorectomy as soon as possible, but it didn't address the main question: Did we want to become parents?

Over time, something changed, and we became less able to speak about it. For years. A part of me longed for the simplicity of my mother and grandmothers' time, when they didn't have access to birth control or choices about whether to have children. It wasn't a question my mother, aunts, and grandmothers had asked themselves. And my generation was the first in my family to have access to our genetic information about hereditary cancer. I had choices. And in that privileged position, I felt the weight of knowledge.

One night in bed, I pointed to the space between our pillows. "Wouldn't it be sweet to have someone small to love?" I asked my husband. I could already smell the head of that baby and feel its warm presence between our bodies. I don't know how to explain it. I felt our baby sleeping between us and I loved this baby so much I was moved to tears. Perhaps this isn't so different from what people feel who actually have babies. Perhaps there is a lot about love that is conjured in our minds.

"Maybe," he said. "Not yet."

I turned my back to him and wiped my tears on my pillowcase, listening to him snore.

*

And then I turned forty. I told Alonso, "We need to make a decision." I waited.

"I want a family," I went on.

"We are a family," he said.

"Two married people are a couple. Not a family."

His expression crumpled as if I'd punched him. "We are," he said. "I'm your family."

I showed him the stack of books that I had been buying since college for this hypothetical child, picture books for bedtime:

Family Pictures / Cuadros de Familia by Carmen Lomas Garza, *Everyone Poops* by Taro Gomi, *Corduroy* by Don Freeman. I had been thinking of my children even when I was a child.

After some time, my husband conceded. "Okay, maybe just one," he said.

*

One of the reasons I had sought therapy after I stopped my grandfather's abuse is because I had read that some survivors of child sexual abuse will become mothers whose own children are abused. As I learned more about my husband's experience as a son, abandoned by his father after his parents divorced, I felt compassion for why he might not want to be a father himself. His father drank too much and partied too hard even after having children. Young Alonso felt his father resented him. There was a time when his father dressed them alike as cowboys and they would get a lot of smiles and attention, but then his father realized that more people were paying attention to the little cowboy than the big one: that was the end of that. Alonso told me about one boyhood birthday, after the divorce, how he waited in the front window for his father, who promised to pick him up to celebrate his birthday. He sat in that window waiting until the morning turned into early afternoon, then evening, then bedtime. His birthday was over. There were worse things his father did. Three words that come to mind to describe his father: alcoholic, womanizer, narcissist. He told Alonso, "You will never make as much money as me," and "Someday you will end up in the gutter where I found you." Alonso feared becoming his father more than anything.

Later in life, I think Alonso's father felt guilty. He sent birthday and Christmas cards to our home and he seemed to know our new address whenever we moved. I recognized Alonso's father's handwriting, and early in our relationship, I would leave out the heavy, thick envelopes on the kitchen counter and watch, in amazement, when Alonso would go right to the trash and throw the envelope away unopened. "What if there's cash in there?" I asked. "Don't you want to know what he wrote to you?" Perhaps his father had recognized the ways he had hurt his son and was asking for forgiveness. I thought something in those envelopes would free Alonso from his childhood pain.

Alonso shrugged and said, "Go ahead if you're so curious." I felt ashamed for being so greedy. One time I did open the envelope, but it was years later, and the envelopes had become noticeably thinner as his father aged. The note inside the greeting card was also spare: *I do love you, Son*. When I learned that Alonso's father was gravely ill, I encouraged Alonso to seek him out—maybe if he had an emotional meeting with his father, like in the movies, something could be healed. But the clock ran out. I hoped that now Alonso would now be free to become a parent. But nothing changed.

*

Removing my ovaries would thrust me immediately into surgical menopause, fifteen years earlier than the age my mother went through the process naturally. I set surgery dates with my gynecologic oncologist and then canceled. Every six months, I went for the ovarian cancer screening appointment: a transvaginal ultrasound, a pelvic exam, and a blood test. I'd traveled to this hospital dozens of times, but now I often drove right past the exit and continued down Storrow Drive. After the appointments—the ones I made it to—I always cried, sometimes openly, in the glass high-rise hallway with beautiful views of Beacon Hill and the State House dome, and sometimes secretly in the gray concrete parking garage where no one could hear me.

It wasn't the risks of surgery or the recovery that scared me. The oophorectomy is a minimally invasive, laparoscopic surgery. I was afraid of suddenly and permanently altering the natural rise and fall of my hormones. I feared what this change would do to who I was. Would I lose my word recall? What does that loss mean for a writer?

There are serious risks to going into menopause at an early age—cardiovascular problems, hot flashes, loss of bone density, and changes in sleep, mood, memory, weight, and energy level. I could partake of hormone replacement therapy, but it would produce a fraction of what my ovaries do. When I brought up those concerns, my doctor replied diplomatically, "We have ways of treating those symptoms, but unfortunately, our options aren't so good once ovarian cancer develops."

I calculated morbid math problems trying to predict which death would be earlier and worse: ovarian cancer or the long-term effects of early menopause. My aunt Ching was diagnosed with ovarian cancer at age sixty-two. I figured I could wait until I was fifty-two to have the surgery and go through menopause naturally, but this was more than a decade past the recommended age for the preventative surgery. My aunt died seven years after her diagnosis. I told myself that maybe I would be one of those mutation carriers who don't develop the disease. But ovarian cancer is called "the silent killer" for a reason. At a conference for people with hereditary cancer, I met a vibrant woman, the founder of a nonprofit for cancer patients, who told me she had ovarian cancer. She seemed energetic and healthy. Two years later, she was dead. Every time I went to my oncologist's waiting room, the ravages of this disease became real. I saw the grief on their faces, what cancer had done to their bodies, and their caretakers helping them walk or pushing their wheelchairs. I felt stupid that I hadn't had the surgery yet. I was rejecting the greatest gift that someone could give me: the chance to change my future.

We decided to freeze embryos, and then I would have my ovaries removed. This would give us a little more time, but not much, to get pregnant. First, we met with a team of physicians, a social worker, and a therapist. We explored pre-implantation genetic diagnosis, which made it possible to select offspring without the BRCA mutation. At forty, I worried that I didn't have enough eggs, but a tech thrust a wand inside me and counted. "A dozen eggs," he said approvingly. I had felt shame in coming to him so late in life and asking for help with such a basic human activity, procreation. But I was relieved to know that I had not asked too late, that I still had eggs. When we met with the doctor after all the tests and consultations were over, it was to start the IVF process in earnest. I was excited.

The doctor leaned across his desk toward Alonso and me. "This is going to be a difficult process, emotionally and physically, and I want to make sure you are both on board with this," he said.

I bounced nervously on my chair, smiling, and then I looked at my husband. He didn't have to say a word. I studied his face for only a moment and then started to weep, loudly. I saw in his expression the look of someone who would do anything for me, including having a child that he did not want. I could see our lives spin out in a flash—how he would uphold his responsibilities as a father, but begrudgingly and without joy. This would be the end of us.

I understood then that motherhood was over for me. My husband loves me, has loved me for almost twenty years, and at that moment, I understood he was only going through with this because I wanted it. I'm old enough to know that love is complex. We don't always get what we want. I was not entitled to motherhood just because I wanted it. I could not subject my husband to this relationship that he did not fully want. And I would not sentence our child, who I imagined I loved already, to a father who was so uncertain. My husband had already been through that with his own father, and it had caused only suffering.

Sometimes I wondered what our lives would have been like had we answered this question earlier, when I was in my twenties, when I was still youthful and pretty, when my breasts were still intact, and I could have met someone else and had a different life in which I was a mother. I'd wonder if I'd married the wrong person. But every time my husband burst through our front door after a run, exuberant and sweaty, I would feel overjoyed that he had returned to me. We shared responsibility. Faced with impossible decisions in which only one of us could win, we let it go and go, until now we were here.

*

I set a date for my oophorectomy and ordered books to read during my recovery. The heaviest one arrived last, *Cook's Illustrated: Cooking for Two*. I paged through shopping tips and meal plans, recipes about how to use half-tomatoes and quarter-onions, partial cans of chicken broth and small cartons of cream until I was rubbing my tears off the pages. I thought about how, for the rest of our lives, we would cook for two until it was time to cook for one.

Another book arrived for me the day after my surgery. It was a picture album of me with my nieces and nephews throughout their lives, some photos taken only hours after they were born. I read the last page and stopped feeling sorry for myself. In bold text, it seemed to shout from the page, "Teetah, we are all your children."

*

When my niece Naomi was twelve, she read me a poem she wrote about me for a school assignment. "My Tita Grace is a very important person in my life," she said. She described me as a "A second mother / The person that plays with you, bakes with you and loves you." I had not expected the love I gave my niece to circle back to me. I realized then that I had been wrong. I was a kind of mother. Sometimes what you long for is what you already have.

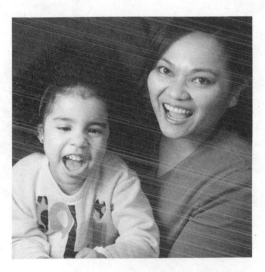

*Grace and her niece Naomi at age 4 after her hair
grew back from chemo. Photo: Alonso Nichols.*

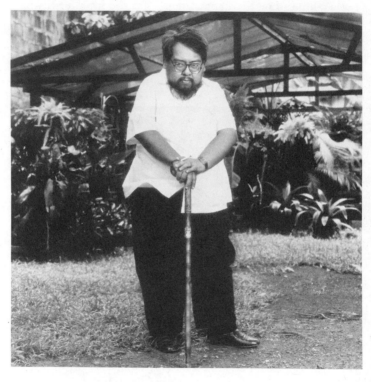

Alfrredo Navarro Salanga in the 1980s. Photo: Wig Tysman.

19

Pasalubong

AS A CHILD, if it weren't for my maternal grandmother's yearly visits from the Philippines, I would not have been certain that such a place existed beyond my family's stories. Mama Lola was as real as the fairy godmother in Cinderella. She swooped in once a year bringing dried watermelon seeds, milk candies, and stories of this fantasyland called Manila, only to vanish without a trace. When Mama Lola noticed that I always had a book in front of my face, she told me about her nephew, Alfrredo Navarro Salanga, who was a prolific writer of journalism, poetry, fiction, criticism, even plays.

"You are becoming like your Tito Freddie," she told me.

I didn't believe Mama Lola. I could not conceive of anyone who looked like me as the author of a book.

Mama Lola told me to write Tito Freddie a letter and she promised to hand-deliver it to him. So, in 1982, at ten years old, I wrote him a letter and forgot about it.

1 October 1984

Dear Grace

It was good to hear from you again – and to learn that you're still going strong and doing well with your music and with your writing. You're twice blessed to be good at both. I never managed to learn how to play a musical instrument – my mother tried to teach me how to play the piano but I was too lazy to keep it up and now I don't even know how to read notes. I do like to listen to music, though, and one of my greatest ambitions still is to write the biography of your great grandfather, Pedro Navarro. I hope your mamalola has been telling you stories of him because I think you have his gift for music. Remember it's a gift and so use it well and treasure it.

Writing, too, is a gift and for that I'm especially glad, being a writer myself. I'm glad you liked <u>Davao Harvest</u>. I've also completed a novel myself which I hope you can get to read when you're a little older – perhaps by the time you're in junior high. In the meantime, I imagine you might be interested in going over some poems that I and four of my friends did. We've dedicated these to the memory of a man I'm sure you've heard about. He was a great man who risked his life and lost it so that we Filipinos can be free. We're not free yet but we will be someday and by then I hope you can come over and pay a visit.

These poems cost us all a great deal of pain because the people who ordered him killed don't like the idea of people thinking him a hero. That may sound strange to you but it is true and that is why you should be thankful that you live in a country where you are free – to write about what you want to and to speak out your mind when you want to. So I hope you do grow up to be a good writer. And do send me a copy of the science fiction novel you're writing. I'll let you know what I think of it after I read it.

My best wishes to you, to your parents and to your mamalola.

Yours affectionaly,

Uncle Freddie
ALFREDO NAVARRO SALANGA

5 Mabuhay Street
East Avenue, Diliman
Quezon City, Philippines

A letter to Grace from Tito Freddie.

The next year, my grandmother returned with a letter tucked into a softcover book titled *Davao Harvest*, by Alfrredo Navarro Salanga. I was amazed. Here was an actual book written by a real writer who was related to me. Back then, I often spent weekends at the public library, but had never encountered a book by a Filipino.

One of the conditions of early childhood is that you must ask for nearly everything that you want. Some objects are out of reach—the ice pops in the freezer—and permission is a constant requirement. Can I play outside? Can I watch TV? Can I have a glass of water? There was always the risk of *No*, and the disappointment, frustration, shame, and longing that accompanied rejection.

The one place I didn't have to ask for permission was in the children's wing at the Ames Free Library. I earned the right to a library card in the first grade by proving I could form the letters to my first and last name on the application. The librarian led me to the picture-book corner where the shelves were my height. There on the red leather bench under the picture window, I found my answers to questions about life and eased my loneliness.

The library was a gift from the Ames family, who made their fortune manufacturing shovels, and I accepted this gift every week. As my mother waited parked out front, I climbed the long walkway to the library's entrance, a low arch trimmed in Longmeadow sandstone, the wooden doors hidden to the left of the entrance on the porch. Later, I learned about the Chinese men who dug the railroad using those Ames shovels. But as a child, all I cared about was getting my books.

I pushed through the dark doors into the library. It was as quiet as a church and just as mysterious. The one toilet in the cellar required a skeleton key and a walk down a narrow spiral staircase, where you were met with the ghostly marble bust of the library's benefactor, Oliver Ames II. Only library staff was allowed to fetch the books from the balcony under the barrel-vaulted ceiling.

My library card was a house key to my true home. Well before I was actually an adult, I was allowed to cross the border into the adult section. When I searched the wooden card catalog, I would always go to the drawer with 959.9 of the Dewey Decimal System and read the name of the place I had come from, which no one had ever heard of.

The summer before I entered college, I worked as a clerk in the library and sat at the glass-topped desk dreaming of who I would become. All that time, I had never thought about all the people who had written the books on the library shelves. The adults I knew were doctors, nurses, teachers, and housewives. And yet, almost a quarter century later, I became a writer. I found stories in that Richardson building early in my life and never stopped looking for more.

*

When it came time for Mama Lola to return to the Philippines, I wrote Tito Freddie another letter where I told him how much I loved his book, even though I was eleven and hadn't been able to make any sense of it.

In October of 1984, my grandmother delivered another

letter from Tito Freddie, the only one that I still possess, along with *In Memoriam: A Poetic Tribute by Five Filipino Poets*. Tito Freddie wrote:

> *These poems cost us all a great deal of pain because the people who ordered him killed don't like the idea of people thinking him a hero. That may sound strange to you but it is true and that is why you should be thankful that you live in a country where you are free—to write about what you want to and to speak out your mind when you want to.*

He was referring to Benigno Aquino Jr, a Filipino senator and long-time political opponent of the Marcos dictatorship who was assassinated in 1983. Aquino had heard rumors that he might be killed if he ever returned to the Philippines, so he invited the press to accompany him on the airplane to Manila so that they might tell his story if he died. There is video footage of the moment before Aquino is shot in the head. He walks through the aisle, steps through the doorway, and meets the bullets. I saw Aquino's clothes displayed in his former home in Newton, Massachusetts, where he had lived in exile. The shirt and pants had stiffened with blood.

I was not yet a teenager, but I was old enough to understand the gravity of what Tito Freddie had written. He picked his words carefully, making me realize how powerful writing could be. Before that day, I had never thought of myself as lucky to live in the U.S. I had taken my freedom of speech for granted.

In the same letter about Aquino, Tito Freddie wrote, "He was a great man who risked his life and lost it so that we Filipinos can be free. We're not free yet but we will be someday, and by then I hope you can come over and pay a visit."

Tito Freddie died before we could meet in person, but his conviction taught me that a writer sets words down, one after the other, which offer new, expansive possibilities.

*

Now, I've kept my promise to my uncle and have returned to the Philippines on a Fulbright fellowship. Midway through my life, I am living in Manila for half a year. My official reason for being here is to work on a research project, but my true motivation is to reconnect with the country that I left as a toddler. What does it mean to have lived most of my life in a different country from the one I had started in?

Once in Manila, I look for signs of Tito Freddie in libraries and bookstores, at his alma mater the Ateneo, at his widow Alice's apartment, and finally at his grave. I read his books; I touch his awards; I flip through hundreds of pages of correspondence, "Thank You" notes that show how generous he was with his time and resources, rejection letters from schools in the U.S. where he had hoped either to study or to teach, and surprisingly warm requests for payment from a bill collector that become sweeter the more time passes.

My aunt Alex once told me that she had read the letters I had written Tito Freddie. "How is that possible?" I asked.

She had seen them on display. I was embarrassed that my

deepest girlhood yearnings had been exhibited. Tita Alex has since passed away, and no one I've asked has ever heard of my letters. I looked, but I didn't find them in the Ateneo archives. Without physical proof, I started to question whether I had even written them—a psychological pattern that I think is intertwined with the immigrant experience. My life in the Philippines had become as believable as a dream.

*

My friend Howie tells me that Freddie "was a writer in the worst of times. He had close friends who were killed by the military; he himself was jailed. He knew that he had gifts that had a higher purpose than just fame and fortune. He gave young writers the gift of his example, time, and attention. He knew that we would grow up and develop into people who could make a difference."

Tito Freddie did not just write poems, novels, short stories, and plays, he also wrote newspaper columns and articles. He was imprisoned for several months during Martial Law for writings critical of the dictatorship. Today, the Philippines is still considered a deadly place to practice journalism, and a bottleneck in the judicial system and a culture of impunity means there is no justice for victims and their families.

*

Across time zones and the globe, Ann messages me the image of my 1984 letter from Tito Freddie while I am visiting Alice, Freddie's widow. We sit together at her dark apartment and she cries as she reads it. In the letter, he describes a project he wants to write, a biography of our common ancestor, Captain Pedro Navarro, and she cries. It's one of many projects he did not have time to complete before his death. After a series of debilitating medical problems, in 1988, Tito Freddie died.

"He wrote beautifully, didn't he?" she says.

Periodically, she pulls a book out from the shelf behind her and reads a favorite poem aloud. Alice does numerology on my birth date and warns me to watch my temper. She explains the second "r" in the spelling of Alfrredo as a decision he made to change his fortune after she read his numbers. Then we share a meal: adobo, home-fermented cabbage, and squares of chocolate from a candy bar for dessert. We talk about the hard times the family faced after Tito Freddie's death. There were medical bills to pay and children to get through school. They moved residences many times and along the way, Alice sold Freddie's book collection, over seven thousand of them, as many as the Philippines had islands, to help pay the bills. A mouse suddenly falls from a hole in the rotting ceiling tile, looks at us, and scampers under a pile of papers.

The only people I've met in the States who know Freddie's work have studied Filipino literature, whereas almost everyone I ask in Manila is not only familiar with his work, but had known him personally. His roots in the literary community were deep.

A few days after visiting Alice, I kneel at Freddie's grave and run my finger across the stone. Although this is my first visit, I've walked past it many times to visit my grandparents and godparents a few rows away. Tito Freddie is buried steps away from the same grandmother who would hand-deliver his letters and books to me in Boston. His epitaph, "The carpenter no longer sings," comes from a poem he wrote after Aquino's assassination. Long after I leave his grave at the cemetery and his papers at the archive, these words continue sounding in my ears.

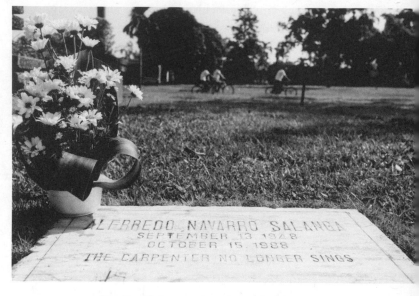

Tito Freddie's gravesite, whose headstone reads,
"The carpenter no longer sings." Photo: Alonso Nichols.

20

A Way of Coming Home

by Alfrredo Navarro Salanga

I think the end came
with his one foot
raised in air—poised
—like an inverted
            benediction

He was stepping down—
isn't that how one goes
into a country from the air?

Hawks and eagles, they too,
land on their feet. But nothing,
nothing was to come out of this,
Neither blessing nor returning.

As the sun touched his crown
it knew. Another door had
                        opened
to welcome him neither

            As a priest
                  nor as bird.

21

Balikbayan

IN THE PHILIPPINES, I am an Amerikano, a returner, a balikbayan. I'm here to learn what it means to be Filipino, but somehow I've only become more American.

It is the last year in the presidency of Noynoy Aquino, whose mother had also been president of the Philippines and whose father Benigno Aquino had been assassinated upon his return. The people I talk to are very hopeful about the future of the Philippines, including my cousin Ronnie. He grew up here and immigrated to the U.S. as an adult, where he spent most of his life. Manong Ronnie returned to the Philippines to retire, but instead became a successful entrepreneur. He is always so excited to talk about the possibilities and potential for growth in the country, encouraging my husband and me to get in early and move here permanently. We consider it. Seriously. We love living in the Philippines, despite its challenges. Only

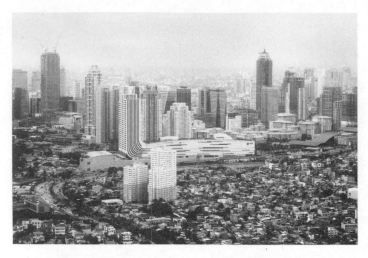

A view of Bonifacio Global City in Metro Manila. Photo: Alonso Nichols.

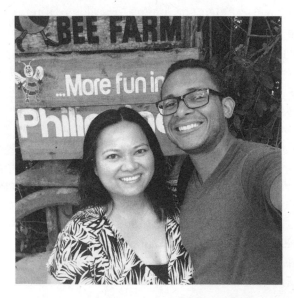

Grace and her husband Alonso at the Bohol Bee Farm on Panglao Island in Bohol, Philippines.

one of us would have to earn a living. On our modest American stipend, we live like the top 1%. The food is easily the best in the world I've ever eaten. We've made close friends fast. Even people we encounter briefly are warm, friendly, and want to connect. It feels good and right to be here. We make inquiries into possible employment and fantasize about what it would mean to call it home. I go on an interview at a call center where I'm told I would be tracked for management, but in order to legally work, first I'll need to sort out my immigration status. I look into becoming a dual citizen.

My husband wants to stay because for the first time he feels the weight of racism lifted from his shoulders. He has not fully realized how heavy and pervasive the burden of living as a Black man in America is until he is in Manila and gets some relief from carrying it. In the Philippines, Alonso is read as American, and this affords him all kinds of benefits and privileges that he has never enjoyed before. He says that being American in the Philippines is what being famous must be like. What it is like to be white. People are always so happy to see him.

At Legaspi Market in Makati, where my husband and I sit for hours on Sunday mornings talking to people in the outdoor market, I meet Erwin Romulo, then editor-in-chief at *Esquire Philippines*. The next week, he gives me a stack of magazines. I stop at the striking black-and-white cover of a man in a jacket with the collar up cradling a large gun, the line "If I were president" underneath his name, "Duterte." This issue is published months before Duterte would announce his run for president, and a full year and a half before he would be inaugurated, before the extrajudicial killing of thousands of people he would set into motion.

In BGC the sidewalks are wide and clean, connecting with crosswalks at every corner. The buildings are white gleaming teeth that bite the clouds. Overhead, cranes pierce the sky, and there is the constant metallic noise of new construction. The poor live on the other side of a wall, and from here it's difficult to see children hauling rocks and garbage unless you stand on tiptoe.

Sometimes, I forget I'm in the Philippines. I feel as though I could be anywhere economically thriving in the States, surrounded as I am by specialty shops for coffee, wine, running shoes, and organic produce. Except that uniformed men with guns stand in the doorways of every bank, condominium, and restaurant. The armed guards promise security, yet I'd never felt so aware of what I could lose: a wallet, a phone, the exact amount of tissue and blood displaced by a bullet.

Things change quickly in BGC. In a fancy restaurant on High Street, Howie tells me that in the 1980s he was detained in solitary confinement for taking photographs of a protest. He waves his hand to indicate that the prison used to be across the street, where a Starbucks and a Lamborghini dealer now stand.

When I ask how long he was detained, Howie says, "Eh, it was only eight days."

"Eight days?"

"There were people there who were held for much longer, or who died," he says.

I imagine that when you're going through it, eight days or a hundred, part of the torture is having no idea how long the imprisonment will last, or if you will survive it.

*

At first I didn't recognize this city transformed from military outpost to consumer center. After college, I'd asked Tita Alex if I could stay with her. She was renting a military officer's house at Fort Bonifacio and I was playing house, but instead of pretending to be a wife and mother, I wanted to role-play a life in the Philippines. Clueless and entitled, I had imposed myself into my aunt's household at the very worst time. She was recovering from a mastectomy and her grandchild, still an infant, was in and out of the hospital with grave difficulties related to Down syndrome. My grandmother, Mama Lola, was also living with my Tita Alex. In her elderly years, Mama Lola had become prone to outbursts of rage and paranoia, accusing the maids of stealing from her, sometimes throwing chairs.

It was August, and sometimes we could not leave the house for days as it rained and rained. To call the maids, my aunt rang a cluster of brass bells, the same ones the altar boy jingled at church when the bread became body. I was in the room one day while her surgical drains were being cleaned, and without thinking, I clutched my own breasts when I saw her wounds, unaware that I was glimpsing my future.

The house was guarded by John and Marsha, a pair of geese named after a couple from a popular Philippine TV sitcom. When tires crunched on the driveway, John and Marsha ran toward the noise, beating their white wings. A maid protected visitors from them by holding an open umbrella between the people's calves and the geese's snapping orange beaks, and at night, John and Marsha huddled in their wooden hut with a door that locked. They listened to the howling of the native dogs that roamed the fields of Fort Bonifacio and the barking of purebred Rottweilers and German shepherds chained outside the homes of military officers. One night, a maid found John squawking and circling the German shepherd that was eating Marsha. The maid swatted the dog with her broom and it fled. Afterward, John died of grief.

One morning, Tita Alex burst into my bedroom and woke me. "Last night the baby died," she cried. "He is with God. He is an angel."

A few years later, my aunt was also gone, from breast cancer, and soon even the military officer's house was gone. Eventually, I return to Fort Bonifacio, but it is now BGC, the body of land transformed so completely and quickly into condos above restaurants, movie theaters, and boutiques that I can barely remember what was here before. I become too distracted by all the fine dining and shopping to locate my grief, to remember what was lost.

*

I often wonder who I would have become if I'd stayed. My parents offer to drop everything to accompany us on the journey. They are worried and afraid. There are reasons they left the Philippines, after all.

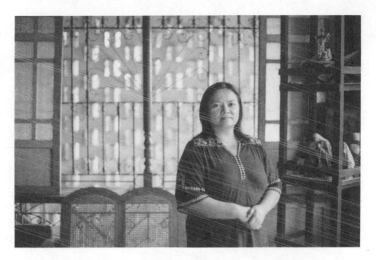

Grace inside the family home in Victoria. Photo: Alonso Nichols.

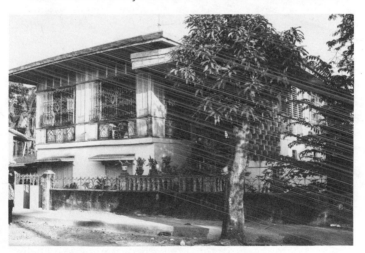

View from across the street of Grace's ancestral
house in Victoria. Photo: Alonso Nichols.

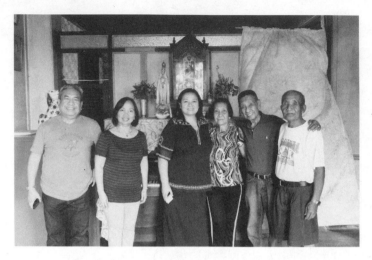

Grace reuniting with relatives in Victoria, from left to right: cousin Ronnie (now deceased) and his wife Becky, Grace, Tita Baby (now deceased), Tito Emil (now deceased), and Baby's husband Toben. Photo: Alonso Nichols.

The plan is to acclimate for a few days in Manila after the 24-hour journey and introduce my husband to our clan. We'll go to our ancestral home in Tarlac, where portraits of people who share my name hang in the municipal buildings. Generations ago, my family enjoyed power as sugar plantation owners, rice processors, and politicians. We'll pose for photos inside the wooden bones of the house, which has been stripped bare over decades, never renovated, and abandoned after everyone left for Manila, and later the United States. When I walk across the living room floor, I am afraid my feet will go through a wooden board. I can see the ground beneath one story below the floorboards where they used to store sacks of rice and sugar to sell. I squint to imagine what was once here during more glorious, prosperous times. I'll keep returning to one photo a year after it's taken, after Tita Baby dies and a few months after that, my cousin Rossini dies, and then eight months after that, his father, my uncle Emilio. They were the keepers of our clan's stories, and I was only able to write down a fraction of these before we ran out of time.

During that first week in Manila, we eat twice as many meals as usual. My relatives play an entertaining game with my husband called *Will the American eat it?* He does. He eats more Filipino foods than I do—*balut*, a hard-boiled egg with an embryonic duck surprise; dinuguan; and all parts of a barbecued chicken: the heads, the feet, even the ass. His relationship to the cuisine is less complicated and less laced with shame than mine. Even now, and even though I know they are delicious, I fear I would have an embarrassing unconscious response if I spooned certain foods into my mouth. We eat fruits—rambutan, *chico*, atis, santol—and desserts—*halo-halo*, *ube halaya, puto, kutsinta, ginataan, puto bumbong*—that never taste the same outside of the Philippines. Filipino foods are influenced by trading and colonization, wars, and invention, by the Americans, the Spanish, the Chinese, and others. Amy Besa, author of *Memories of Philippine Kitchens*, and owner of the Purple Yam, describes our cuisine as "everything that grows in our environment, and what people do to it to eat and survive."

My favorite fruit in the world is the Philippine mango. It is exquisite, and even when I find it outside of the islands, I am disappointed. We pass a mango grove in Bohol, and each fruit wears a jacket made of newspaper to protect it from pests and temperature changes. I think of the person who made the clothes and dressed the fruit so gently that it didn't fall from the branch. I savor every bite. My mother complains that my father is eating too much. "Why does he have to eat every hour?" Even my husband cannot keep up with my father's appetite. I ask my mother to lay off. There are some things that you can only eat in Manila.

Every food my parents eat comes with a story they don't remember until they've chewed the memory in their mouths. My father tells us that as a boy, he used to eat these same ice cream sandwiches on the street, a scoop of purple *ube* ice cream between two pieces of soft white bread. My mother, her mouth greasy with orange fat, says she hasn't eaten these tiny mud crabs since she was a little girl, and for a moment, I can see that girl, that boy, who will eventually become my parents.

Most of our time is spent walking through the crowded shopping centers and sitting in the crawling traffic. Children in rags, with the faces of my nieces and nephews, appear at our windows, begging. "Knock on the window," I was told. "That will make them go away." One time in traffic I watched orange flames shoot from the front of a city bus and move toward the back, where passengers were jumping out onto the highway overpass. I was scared that someone would burn alive, but when I watched the news that night, there were no fatalities.

There are so many malls and super mega malls in Manila that some argue that the city itself is one giant mall. It is the perfect place to meet people—if the other party is delayed by traffic, which happens always and sometimes for hours, you can wander around air-conditioned stores or go to a movie. The patrons seem happy, happier than Americans I've seen at malls back home. Early on in our trip, I stand alone at a balcony inside a mall, levels above and below, watching uniformed students and workers ride up and down the jam-packed escalators. There are so many Filipinos walking by me, more than I've ever seen. I'm not used to being around so many people who look familiar. I almost chase a woman, certain she is my aunt Rose, until I remember that I attended her funeral years ago in California.

My father appears next to me with another bag of something to eat and offers me some. "I can't, Dad. I'm still so full," I say.

We stand arm to arm. I'm dizzy with jetlag and the heat and the dueling Whitney Houston songs. I lean toward my father. Our arms are warm in such close proximity, but neither of us moves away. This is the most physical affection I've shared with him since we danced at my wedding. I let my head lean near his shoulder, but don't make contact. We are quiet together, mesmerized by the people constantly in motion.

I try to find a version of myself in the crowd. In my alternate Philippines life, would I already be the mother to a soccer team-sized brood of children? Would I still be a writer? Sometimes I think I would have been happier in the Philippines, and sometimes I wonder if I would already be dead. My lungs don't do well with the city's pollution, and I've ended up in a Manila emergency room more than once with difficulty breathing. Or perhaps cancer would have consumed me by now and made my theoretical Filipino family widowed and motherless. Even if the genetic test for hereditary breast and ovarian cancer had been accessible to me in the Philippines, I doubt I would have had the preventive surgeries in time.

During that trip, when I find myself receiving medical care for something unrelated at one of the finest hospitals in the Philippines, the examining physician is curious about my reconstructed breast mounds. In the interest of science and cultural exchange, I answer his questions and lift my shirt. "You didn't have breast cancer, but you had a mastectomy?" he asks.

"It's what's recommended for women with the BRCA mutation," I explain. I asked if he had heard of hereditary breast and ovarian cancer and genetic testing.

He touches my scars without gloves and then scolds me. "What does your husband think of this mutilation? You should have waited," he says. "God has a plan."

I should have waited for cancer to take root in my body? As an older male doctor, he is technically higher in status, but I don't hide my contempt. "I did the right thing," I tell him. "I'm certain of it. And as for my husband, he prefers me alive."

As my father and I stand together on the mall bridge, I have a thought. Maybe it's that I'm in a new place and it feels possible to act in a new way. I don't talk myself out of speaking. "I'm really glad you and Mom took the time to bring us to Manila. I don't think we could have navigated it as well without you. We don't have the language skills. We don't know the culture." I feel my father's body sway forward and back.

"Of course," he says.

I've never expressed myself so directly to my father, and I've certainly never shown my appreciation so baldly. From my childhood years, I'd learned to expect humiliation and to fear being wounded at exactly the moment when I'm the most vulnerable. Except to my nieces and nephews, whom I shower with love unabashedly, I am reticent to express how I feel. But being back in my first home seems to give me the courage to speak what is in my heart. "Dad, I've never told you this before, but I want to thank you for bringing us to America. I'm not saying that I would have had a bad life in the Philippines. Just a different one."

He's surprised, turning his body to look at me. I wonder if in that moment he's remembering my pain. He responds in a gentle voice, a rare timbre that I have not heard since I was a young girl, when I felt loveable, before his father ruined my life. Once a year on my birthday, I still feel this way, loved and free. In my father's voice, I hear his potential to be endlessly compassionate and insightful, someone capable of expressing affection and love without fear. My father isn't able to be this person very often. He's been shaped by generations of trauma and suffers in ways I recognize.

*

My father also remembers this moment between us, but his memory places us in a different time and setting. His version of the story surprises me. In it, I am younger and much more effusive. I don't recognize myself in my father's recollection. He is more heroic. At first, when he shares his remembrance,

I argue with him. "Dad, I remember very clearly that we were standing on the balcony at the mall, and you were eating." His face falls and I stop. He is as certain of his memory as I am of mine. What does it matter whether we were in the mall or in the van? What matters most is that I thanked my father and he heard me. In his telling, he reveals his deepest wishes for our relationship, and somehow, this wish has become his memory. I wonder how often my father has replayed this moment to himself, and what it has helped him bear.

In his version, we're in Manila; he is sitting in the front passenger seat of the van and I'm behind him, napping. We're in traffic. Suddenly, I wake from a deep sleep. I lunge forward and press myself against the back of my father's seat, wrapping my arms around his chest. He's surprised, but he puts his hands on mine. I speak in a loud voice, he tells me, so loud that everyone in the van can hear me, even over the music, the air-conditioning, and the street noise. "Daddy!" I say. "Thank you for taking us to America. I love you so very much."

ACKNOWLEDGMENTS

My first note of appreciation is for the judges of the Restless Books Prize for New Immigrant Writing, Anjali Singh and Ilan Stavans, who created a space for me on the bookshelf. I am grateful for your vision, mission, and vigorous support of writers like me.

Thank you to the entire Restless Books team, especially my editor Nathan Rostron, who read my work carefully, tirelessly, and compassionately. You are a remarkable editor and a kind soul. Thank you to Strick & Williams for the stunning cover. With gratitude to my agent, Jenni Ferrari-Adler, for your enthusiastic support and wise counsel.

I have loved books since I earned my first public library card by proving that I could write my name, first and last, print and cursive. That was a long time ago. A lifetime of people helped me become a writer, but there are too many to name here so I will describe you: You put books in my hands; you recommended authors of color who I did not learn about in school: Carlos Bulosan, Jessica Hagedorn, Sandra Cisneros, Maxine Hong Kingston, Lynda Barry, Toni Cade Bambara, and countless others. Seeing myself reflected in other writers of color made it possible for me to imagine that I could write about my reality. You shared your story with me as a fellow survivor or a previvor. You expressed what my work means to you. You gave me feedback; you shared my writing; you invited me to speak to your students and book clubs; you gave me paid work so that I could continue my unpaid work; you encouraged me in tiny and big ways to keep writing even when I was certain that no one would want my stories, and for that, I am eternally grateful. Thank you to journalists for your courageous reporting and commitment to finding the truth. Your work changed my life, especially the *Boston Globe*'s Spotlight team.

I am grateful to librarians, archivists, and funders of public libraries, especially the Ames Free Library, Tufts University Libraries, the Library and Research Center of the Missouri Historical Society, the Filipinas Heritage Library, the University Archives of Ateneo de Manila University, and many other university and local libraries where I accessed materials and worked for hours in peaceful spaces that revere the written word. With appreciation to the National Archives and Records Administration for the documents that came from my FOIA request. I received vital encouragement and resources at crucial times in my writing life from the Massachusetts Cultural Council, the Somerville Arts Council, the Center for Study of Women in Society at the University of Oregon, the Women's National Book Association, the Tufts Part-time Faculty Professional Development Fund, and other grants, large and small. I wish to acknowledge the support of artist residencies and summer workshops such as the Writer's Room of Boston, Hedgebrook, Ragdale, the Dune Shacks of the Provincetown Community Compact, Wellspring House, Provincetown Fine Arts Work Center, Voices of Our Nation, and the Community of Writers at Squaw Valley. I am grateful for informal writing residencies, such as the magical yellow house of Finn and Henriette Lazaridis, Tita Alex's spare bedroom, and the many coffee shops where I overstayed my welcome.

This book was made possible through the support of the Fulbright Scholar Program and the Philippine American Educational Foundation. Thank you to Luisa Igloria, for connecting me to my Fulbright mentor, Isagani Cruz, who introduced me to essential people as well as the best Manila lunch spots. A halo-halo for fellow Fulbrighters Joseph Legaspi and Jason Reblando, who processed this complicated experience with me in real time, and a mango shake for Natalie Masuoka, Gordon Au, John Diaz, Sharon Crame, and Gus Reblando for being there. I arrived too late to meet my childhood pen pal, Alfrredo Navarro Salanga, but I am grateful for his poems and the time I spent with his widow, Alice, and his daughter, Elyrah Salanga-Torralba. Thank you to Tito Freddie's friends, especially Howie Severino, Krip Yuson, and Melvyn Calderon for sharing their memories, and Wig Tysman for the photo. With deep gratitude to the strangers I shared conversations with in the Philippines and the friends I made in Manila, especially Laurel Fantauzzo, Sunshine Lichauco De Leon, Bong Albar, Tita Valderama, Nadine Sarreal, and the great Howie Severino, who invited us along on his adventures and whose friendship continues to give us unexpected gifts.

Ako ay lubos na nagpapasalamat sa lahat ng mga tumulong para sa publikasyon ng aking libro. May maraming salamat sa mga pamilya, especially the Gamalinda and Talusan clans, and my second mom, Tita Aida. Special gratitude to those relatives who fed me, in more ways than one, during my Fulbright, but died before this book was published. Rest in peace Alice Salanga, Al Peter Salanga, Tita Baby, Cornelio Talusan, Rossini Gamalinda, and Emilio Navarro Gamalinda. Aileen says you have already seen this book. If so, I hope I've made you proud.

I am grateful to fellow students and teachers from elementary school through graduate school. Each of you helped me become the writer and teacher I am today. Thank you to N. V. M. Gonzalez, Geoffrey Wolff, Michelle Latiolais, Dorianne Laux, Ehud Havazelet, Garrett Hongo, Debra Gwartney, Jenna Blum, and so many other writers who taught me crucial lessons when I needed them. Thank you to recent teachers and students of online writing courses from the Writers Studio, Creative Nonfiction, GrubStreet, and especially Lidia Yuknavitch's Corporeal Writing for helping me find the backbone of this book.

Thank you to the staff, faculty, friends, and my students at GrubStreet, the best literary community around. Special thanks to founder, Eve Bridburg, and to Christopher Castellani for inviting me into GrubStreet in the first place.

I am grateful for the many folks, more than I can name, at Tufts University who supported my work, first as a student and later, as a faculty member. With appreciation to Jonathan Strong, Modhumita Roy, Lynn Stevens, Jonathan Wilson, Lisa Coleman, Ruth Hsiao, Peggy Barrett, Melody Komyerov, Mindy Nierenberg, Shirley Mark, Sherri Sklarwitz, Sara Allred, Jessye Crowe-Rothstein, Francie Chew, Yolanda King, Jean Wu, James Glaser, Louise Dunlap, Christina Sharpe, and Linell Yugawa.

Thank you to all of my Tufts students, with special recognition to my first generation to college, low income, immigrant, undocumented, LGBTQ, and POC students who inspire me to fight, but also to dream. I hope my story makes a space for you to tell yours.

Thank you to Filipino readers, wherever you are in the world. I am indebted to the Boston Filipino American Book Club, especially the founder Bren Bataclan, whose project of buying and reading new books by living Filipino American writers reminded me constantly that I had eager readers waiting for my book. Thank you to the FLIPS listserv, the Filipino American National Historical Society, the Asian American Writers Workshop, Voices of Our Nation, and other organizations who center our stories.

I am grateful for friends who asked all the right questions and helped me through crucial times: Meg DeSantis, Alan Liska, Rivka Simmons, Kristen Rice, Julie Merrill, Pamela Goldstein, Suzan Wolpow, Regis Donovan, Sarah Seitz, Demetra Barlas, Sue Friedman, Pagan Kennedy, Marie Lee, Michelle Seaton, Vicki Forman, Luke Rigas, Jennifer Goulart, Len Farnham, Todd Larson, Erin Leiman, Tom Elliott, and especially, Marcia Weiss for your compassion and for seeing what I could not. Jeffrey Rubin answered my immigration questions almost instantly. I am astounded by the generosity of those who volunteered to read this manuscript, Nathaniel Tran, Marcia Weiss, Meredith Talusan, Gilmore Tamny, Beth Castrodale, Marie Lee, Joanne Diaz, Roslyn Talusan, and others. With gratitude to Javed Rezayee, Cheryl Hamilton, and others in the storytelling community who helped me find the green station wagon story. Deep appreciation to editors who published pieces which became portions of this book, especially David Brittan, John Wolfson, Karen Bailey, Taylor McNeil, Sarge Lacuesta, Genevieve Rajewski, Nicole Chung, Jennifer Barber, Dinty W. Moore, Hattie Fletcher, Lee Gutkind, Richard Hoffman, Lee Hope, Greg Harris, Roxane Gay, and other editors.

Thank you to all of my previous writing groups, especially 17 Syllables, and to friends who helped me with early drafts: Audrey Schulman, Mary Sullivan Walsh, Sally Bunch, Beth Castrodale, Sabina Chen, and Gilmore Tamny, sisters of my heart. Thank you Dr. Mary Talusan Lacanlale for your work on the PC Band. I am grateful to the many people sat across from me on writing dates, especially Natalie Masuoka for the years of Fridays we spent together at Starbucks laughing, talking, and keeping each other honest so that we could write our books. My gratitude and appreciation to the writing group who changed everything for me, the Chunky Monkeys: Christopher Castellani, Chip Cheek, Calvin Hennick, Jennifer De Leon, Sonya Larson, Alex Marzano-Lesnevich, Celeste Ng, Whitney Scharer, Adam Stumacher, and Becky Tuch. Soon our books will fill a shelf.

Without Joanne Diaz, there simply would be no book. Only a poet as attentive to language and image as Joanne could sit beside me one morning in a BGC Starbucks, both of us shivering in the refrigerator-cold climate, amidst my pile of essays and despair, and proclaim, "This is a book called *The Body Papers*." Thank you, Joanne, for believing that I am a better person than I think I am. You inspire me to be that better person.

I have the greatest in-laws in the world. Thank you for making me "Teetah" and loving me so fiercely. My mother-in-law, Mary Ann Nichols, inspires me with her dignity and tells the best stories.

It is impossible to convey my profound love and appreciation to my husband, Alonso Nichols. You believed in me and loved me through ups and downs, from far away and close up. Every time I was close to giving up, your love and conviction kept me going just a little longer.

With deep appreciation and gratitude to my parents and siblings who encouraged my storytelling with good humor, enthusiasm, and respect in spite of everything. This book is my love letter to you. *Mahal kita.*

ABOUT THE AUTHOR

GRACE TALUSAN was born in the Philippines and raised in New England. She graduated from Tufts University and the MFA Program in Writing at UC Irvine. She is the recipient of a U.S. Fulbright Fellowship to the Philippines and an Artist Fellowship Award from the Massachusetts Cultural Council. Grace teaches the Essay Incubator at GrubStreet and courses in the Jonathan M Tisch College of Civic Life at Tufts University. She is the Fannie Hurst Writer-in-Residence at Brandeis University for 2019–2021.

RESTLESS BOOKS is an independent, nonprofit publisher devoted to championing essential voices from around the world, whose stories speak to us across linguistic and cultural borders. We seek extraordinary international literature that feeds our restlessness: our hunger for new perspectives, passion for other cultures and languages, and eagerness to explore beyond the confines of the familiar. Our books—fiction, narrative nonfiction, journalism, memoirs, travel writing, and young people's literature—offer readers an expanded understanding of a changing world.